Handbook of

EEG
INTERPRETATION

D1375512

Handbook of
EEG
INTERPRETATION

William O. Tatum, IV, DO

Section Chief, Department of Neurology, Tampa General Hospital
Clinical Professor, Department of Neurology, University of South Florida
Tampa, Florida

Aatif M. Husain, MD

Associate Professor, Department of Medicine (Neurology), Duke University Medical Center
Director, Neurodiagnostic Center, Veterans Affairs Medical Center
Durham, North Carolina

Selim R. Benbadis, MD

Director, Comprehensive Epilepsy Program, Tampa General Hospital
Professor, Departments of Neurology and Neurosurgery, University of South Florida
Tampa, Florida

Peter W. Kaplan, MB, FRCP

Director, Epilepsy and EEG, Johns Hopkins Bayview Medical Center
Professor, Department of Neurology, Johns Hopkins University School of Medicine
Baltimore, Maryland

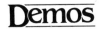

Acquisitions Editor: R. Craig Percy
Developmental Editor: Richard Johnson
Cover Designer: Steve Pisano
Indexer: Joann Woy
Compositor: Patricia Wallenburg
Printer: Victor Graphics

Visit our website at www.demosmedpub.com

Library of Congress Cataloging-in-Publication Data
Handbook of EEG interpretation / William O. Tatum IV ... [et al.].
   p. ; cm.
Includes bibliographical references and index.
ISBN-13: 978-1-933864-11-2 (pbk. : alk. paper)
ISBN-10: 1-933864-11-7 (pbk. : alk. paper)
  1. Electroencephalography—Handbooks, manuals, etc.   I. Tatum, William O.
[DNLM: 1. Electroencephalography—methods—Handbooks. WL 39 H23657 2007]
RC386.6.E43H36 2007
616.8'047547—dc22

                                                              2007022376

Medicine is an ever-changing science undergoing continual development. Research and
clinical experience are continually expanding our knowledge, in particular our knowledge
of proper treatment and drug therapy. The authors, editors, and publisher have made
every effort to ensure that all information in this book is in accordance with the state of
knowledge at the time of production of the book.

Nevertheless, this does not imply or express any guarantee or responsibility on the part of
the authors, editors, or publisher with respect to any dosage instructions and forms of
application stated in the book. Every reader should examine carefully the package inserts
accompanying each drug and check with a his physician or specialist whether the dosage
schedules mentioned therein or the contraindications stated by the manufacturer differ
from the statements made in this book. Such examination is particularly important with
drugs that are either rarely used or have been newly released on the market. Every dosage
schedule or every form of application used is entirely at the reader's own risk and responsibility. The editors and publisher welcome any reader to report to the publisher any dis-
crepancies or inaccuracies noticed.

Made in the United States of America

07 08 09 10   5 4 3 2 1

This book is dedicated to our families,
our fine colleagues interested in EEG,
our friends in the field of EEG technology,
and especially our patients.

CONTENTS

PREFACE

In any field of medicine, the best quality of care is proportional to the knowledge of the practitioner. In the case of electroencephalography (EEG), this knowledge is a function of experience and, for most, that experience is a function of exposure. Therefore, within the chapters outlined in this book, exposure to the functional uses of EEG is provided not as a sole representation, but rather as a supplement to clinical experience. Essential, "bottom-line" information is provided to help readers with the challenges of EEG interpretation. Historically, on-the-job training, usually in a one-on-one setting, has been the standard by which most neophyte electroencephalographers acquire the exposure from those who are more senior in experience and knowledge. While much of these same methods continue to be used in large university settings to educate neurologists and neurophysiologists, the role of the internet and classroom educational experiences are not capable of being retained "at the bedside" during encounters with real-life EEG recordings. Thus, *Handbook of EEG Interpretation* is intended to fill a void by providing quick and easy access to key topics in EEG in the hopes of ultimately providing better patient care. Correctly identifying normal and abnormal EEGs brings important information to the clinician taking care of patients. Epileptiform abnormalities and identification of ictal EEG patterns make the interpretation of the EEG the ideal study for evaluating patients with seizures or suspected epilepsy. Patterns of special significance underlie features that appear often during states of stupor or coma. Chapters on sleep and neurointensive and intraoperative monitoring add useful information to complete the handbook for clinicians that would benefit from quick and easy pattern recognition.

To properly preface this work, it must first be understood that the clinical interpretation of EEG is one art within the vast field of clinical neurophysiology. Many excellent works have served to advance our knowledge of EEG, yet are unable to be represented within a portable handbook. The intent for the reader is to provide a "bullet" of information with a graphic representation of the principal features in EEG, and thus provide a quick neurophysiology reference that is so crucial during the bedside interpretation of one's "brainwaves." We have written *Handbook of EEG Interpretation* to fit into the lab coat pockets of *all* health care professionals who need access to quick, reliable EEG information: neurologists, other physicians, and other health care providers; young and old; and new and learned within the field in the hope of providing a portable service to our colleagues and patients. With the unique characteristics provided by EEG, we can only expect that, as our knowledge base grows within the field of neurophysiology, the application of EEG within other areas of medicine will grow and have a more widespread application in the future.

William O. Tatum, IV, DO
Aatif M. Husain, MD
Selim R. Benbadis, MD
Peter W. Kaplan, MD

DKWILY

Handbook of

EEG

INTERPRETATION

Normal EEG

WILLIAM O. TATUM, IV

The value of understanding the normal EEG lies in developing the foundation to provide a clinical basis for identifying abnormality. Knowledge of normal waveform variations, variants of normal that are of uncertain significance, and fluctuations of normal EEG throughout the lifecycle from youth to the aged are essential to provide an accurate impression for clinical interpretation. When abnormality is in doubt, a conservative impression of "normal" is proper.

The electroencephalogram (EEG) is a unique and valuable measure of the brain's electrical function. It is a graphic display of a difference in voltages from two sites of brain function recorded over time. Electroencephalography (EEG) involves the study of recording these electrical signals that are generated by the brain. Extracranial EEG provides a broad survey of the electrocerebral activity throughout both hemispheres of the brain. Intracranial EEG provides focused EEG recording directly from the brain through surgically implanted electrodes that are targeted at specific regions of the brain. Information about a diffuse or focal cerebral dysfunction, the presence of interictal epileptiform discharges (IEDs), or patterns of special significance may be revealed. For the successful interpretation of an abnormal EEG, one must first understand the criteria necessary to define normal patterns. While a normal EEG does not exclude a clinical diagnosis (i.e., epilepsy), an abnormal finding on EEG may be supportive of a diagnosis (i.e., in epilepsy), be indicative of cerebral dysfunction (i.e., focal or generalized slowing), or have nothing to do with the reason that the study was performed (i.e., in headache). It is the clinical application of the EEG findings that imparts the utility of EEG.

BASIC PHYSIOLOGY OF
CEREBRAL POTENTIALS

The origin of cerebral potentials is based upon the intrinsic electrophysiological properties of the nervous system. Identifying the generator source(s) and electrical field(s) of propagation are the basis for recognizing electrographic patterns that underly the expression of the "brain waves" as normal or abnormal. Most routine EEGs recorded at the surface of the scalp represent pooled electrical activity generated by large numbers of neurons.

Electrical signals are created when electrical charges move within the central nervous system. Neural function is normally maintained by *ionic gradients* established by neuronal membranes. Sufficient duration and length of small amounts (in microvolts) of electrical currents of cerebral activity are required to be amplified and displayed for interpretation. A *resting (diffusion) membrane potential* normally exists through the efflux of positive-charged (potassium) ions maintaining an *electrochemical equilibrium* of –75 mV. With *depolarization*, an influx of positive-charged (sodium) ions that exceeds the normal electrochemical resting state occurs. Channel opening within the lipid bilayer is via a voltage-dependent mechanism, and closure is time dependent. Conduction to adjacent portions of the nerve cell membranes results in an action potential when the depolarization threshold is exceeded. However, it is the *synaptic potentials* that are the most important source of the extracellular current flow that produces potentials in the EEG. *Excitatory postsynaptic potentials* (EPPs) flow inwardly (extracellular to intracellular) to other parts of the cell (*sinks*) via sodium or calcium ions. *Inhibitory post-synaptic potentials* (IPPs) flow outwardly (intracellular to extracellular) in the opposite direction (*source*), and involve chloride or potassium ions. These summed potentials are longer in duration than action potentials and are responsible for most of the EEG waveforms. The brainstem and thalamus serve as subcortical generators to synchronize populations of neocortical neurons in both normal (i.e., sleep elements) and in abnormal situations (i.e., generalized spike-and-wave complexes).

Volume conduction characterizes the process of current flow from the brain generator and recording electrode.

Layers of cortical neurons are the main source of the EEG. *Pyramidal cells* are the major contributor of the synaptic potentials that make up EEG (Figure 1.1A). These neurons are arranged in a perpendicular orientation to the cortical surface from *layers III*, *IV*, and *VI*. Volumes large enough to allow measurement at the surface of the scalp require areas that are >6 cm^2 , although probably >10 cm^2 are required for most IEDs to appear on the scalp EEG because of the attenuating properties incurred by the skull. All generators have both a positive and negative pole that function as a *dipole* (Figure 1.1B). The EEG displays the continuous and changing voltage fields varying with different locations on the scalp.

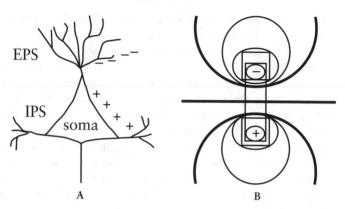

FIGURE 1.1. (A) A pyramidal cell with excitatory postsynaptic potentials and inhibitory postsynaptic potentials. (B) Dipole depicting a field of charge separation.

Scalp EEG recording displays the difference in electrical potentials between two different sites on the head overlying cerebral cortex that is closest to the recording electrode. During routine use, electrical potentials are acquired indirectly from the scalp surface and incorporate waveform analyses of frequency, voltage, morphology, and topography. However, most of the human cortex is buried deep beneath the scalp surface, and additionally represents a two-dimensional projection of a three-dimensional source, presenting a problem for generator localization in scalp EEG. Furthermore, the waveforms that are recorded from the scalp represent *pooled synchronous activity* from large populations of neurons that create the cortical potentials and may not represent small interictal or ictal sources.

Initial one-channel EEG recordings in the late 1920s have evolved to sophisticated digital-based computerized recording devices. From the patient scalp, electrodes conduct electrical potentials to an *electrode box* (jackbox). Thereafter, a montage selector permits EEG signals to pass through amplifiers before filtering and ancillary controls regulate the signal output. Data display follows acquisition and processing and has a wide variety of data presentation for EEG interpretation. Electrode placement has been standardized by an international 10–20 system that uses anatomical landmarks on the skull. These sites are then subdivided by intervals of 10% to 20% and to designate the site where an electrode will be placed. A minimum of 21 electrodes are recommended for clinical study, although digital EEG now has the capability for a greater number. During infant EEG recordings, fewer electrodes are used depending upon age and head size. A newer modified combinatorial electrode system uses electrode placement with more closely spaced electrodes in a 10–10 system (Figure 1.2). The designations; Fp (frontopolar), F (frontal), T (temporal), O (occipital), C (central), and P (parietal) are utilized in the 10–20 system. Subsequently, numbers combined following the letters for location reflect either the left (odd numbers) or right (even numbers) hemisphere of electrode placement. The "z" designation reflects midline placement (i.e., Cz = central midline). In the 10–10 system, lower numbers in their positions reflect locations closer to the midline, and T3/T4 become T7/T8, while T5/T6 become P7/P8. Electrode impedances should be maintained between 100 and 5000 ohms. Special electrodes may also be added such as sphenoidal, true temporal, or frontotemporal electrodes. Most are employed for the purpose of delineating temporal localization. True temporal electrodes (designated T1 and T2) are placed to help distinguish anterior temporal or posterior inferior frontal location not delineated by the F7 or F8 positions. Combining the 10–20 system with electrodes from the 10–10 system may be most practical for routine clinical use as additional electrodes become desired. Colloidion is a compound used to secure electrodes during prolonged recording techniques such as during video-EEG or ambulatory monitoring. Paste used for routine recordings is more temporary. Subdermal electrodes are used when other recording techniques are not feasible such as in the operating room and intensive care unit.

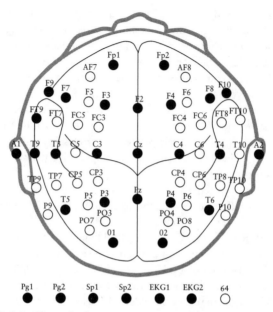

FIGURE 1.2. Electrode placements systems use either a 10-20 system (black circles) or modified combinatorial system with 10-10 electrode placement (black circles + white circles).

Other added electrodes may include electrocardiogram (EKG) (recommended with every EEG), eye movement monitors, electromyogram (EMG), and extracerebral electrodes to aid in artifact differentiation, or with sleep staging in the case of eye lead monitors. Respiratory monitors may also be important if respiratory problems are identified.

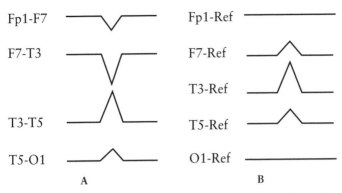

FIGURE 1.3. (A) Bipolar montage demonstrating phase reversal and (B) referential montage demonstrating absolute voltage.

The electrical "map" obtained from the spatial array of recording electrodes used is the montage. Several montages are used throughout a 20- to 30-minute routine EEG recording. Every routine EEG should include at least one montage using a longitudinal bipolar, reference, and traverse bipolar montage (Figures 1.3 and 1.4). A reference montage uses an active electrode site as the initial input, and then at least one "neutral" electrode to depict absolute voltage through amplitude measurement that is commensurate with the area of maximal electronegativity or postivity (Figure 1.3B). A midline reference electrode (i.e., Pz), may be useful for lateralizing temporal recordings. However, two references (i.e., ipsilateral ear reference) and may be useful for more generalized discharges. Even multiple "averaged" sites of reference (or Laplacian montages for very focal recordings) may be useful for localized discharges. Bipolar montages may be arranged in many different spatial formats including longitudinally, transverse fashion, or in a circumferential pattern. The longitudinal bipolar (also called "double banana") is frequently represented throughout this text. An anterior to posterior temporal and central connecting chain of electrodes arranged left alternating with right-sided placement is a typical array. Bipolar montages compare active electrodes sites adjacent to each other and signify absolute electrographic sites of maximal negativity (or positivity) by phase reversals (Figure 1.3A).

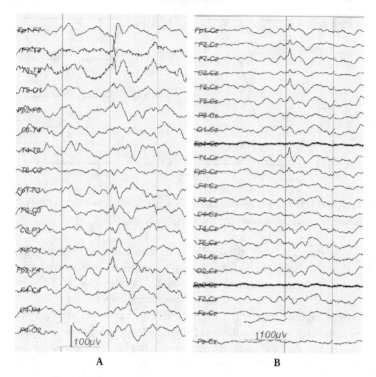

FIGURE 1.4. EEG demonstrating bipolar (A) and reference (B) montages to illustrate a left anterior temporal sharp wave.

EEG	Electrode 1	Electrode 2
Negative	Up	Down
Positive	Down	Up

FIGURE 1.5. The rules governing polarity and convention relative to "pen" deflection. When input 1 is negative the deflection is up.

By convention, when the voltage difference between electrode 1 is more negative than electrode 2, deflection of the waveform is *up*. Recordings are usually performed with a visual display of 30 mm/sec (slower with sleep studies), amplifier sensitivities of 7 ÌV/mm, and filter settings of 1 to 70 Hz. Reducing the low filter settings promotes slower frequency representation, while reducing high filter settings decrease high frequency. A narrow band reduction is possible using a notched filter setting to limit 60-Hz interference (50-Hz in the UK). Proprietary software offers digital seizure and spike detection capabilities for digital EEG systems that are commercially available for both routine and prolonged EEG monitoring. This section will encompass patterns of cerebral and extracerebral origin, as well as patterns of uncertain significance to illustrate the range of normal EEGs encountered in clinical practice.

EXTRACEREBRAL ARTIFACTS

Recording electrical activity from the brain is subject to noncerebral interference. Various generators of nonphysiological and physiological artifacts may deceive the interpreter to believe that the apparent sources are abnormal or epileptiform. When in doubt, it is incumbent upon the EEG interpreter to assume that the source is an artifact until proven otherwise.

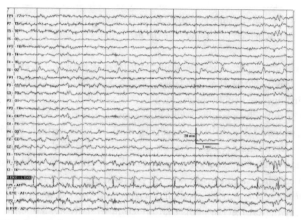

FIGURE 1.6. Pulse artifact mimicking PLEDs at the T6 derivation. Note the 1:1 relationship to the EKG and field limited to a single electrode.

The EKG should be monitored during EEG to provide information about the relationship between the heart and the brain. The QRS complex of the EKG represents the largest deflection and often confers artifact. An EKG artifact may appear simultaneously with prominent QRS complexes seen in several channels. Ballistocardiographic potentials reveal a movement artifact that is time locked to the EKG. In the example above, pulse artifact is seen that is usually seen in a single channel as a periodic slow wave. It occurs when an electrode is in a position that is near an artery. There is a discrete time-locked 1:1 relationship between the heat rate and the periodic potential created by the pulse to produce an artifact on the EEG.

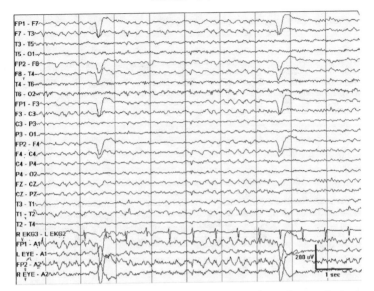

FIGURE 1.7. Eye movement monitors demonstrating the *in-phase* cerebral origin of the diffusely slow background in this awake patient, and the *out-of-phase* movement of the eye blink artifacts during seconds 3 and 8.

An eye blink artifact seen in the EEG (see above) is generated by the electrical potential produced by vertical movement of the eye. Normally, the eye functions as an electrical dipole with a relative positivity of the cornea compared to the retina. The potential created is a DC potential of higher amplitude (mV) than the amplitude produced by the brain (μV). The artifact is produced in the electrodes around the eye (FP1/2) during vertical eye movements. With an eye blink, the cornea rolls up with resultant positivity in the FP1/2 electrodes relative to the F3/4 electrodes and creates a downward deflection during the normal Bell's phenomenon. Electrodes recording above and below the eye will help to distinguish the brain as the "generator" (same polarity is every channel) from an artifact (opposite polarity in electrode sites above and below the eye).

11

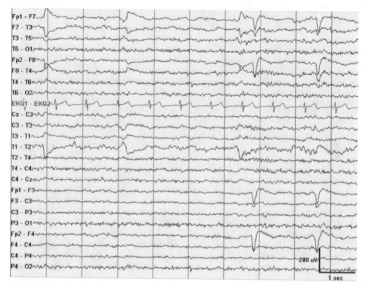

FIGURE 1.8. Artifact from three horizontal eye movements (looking left) followed by two vertical eye blinks.

The presence of a vertical eye blink artifact helps define the state of the patient as being awake. During drowsiness, slow rolling (lateral) eye movements are similarly helpful. Lateral eye movements are usually easily recognized because they create phase reversals in the anterior temporal derivations that are of opposite polarity on opposite sides of the scalp EEG. When the eyes move to the left yielding a positive phase reversal in F7 due to the cornea polarity, the homologous F8 electrode site demonstrates a negative phase reversal from the retina. Note the two lateral eye movements at the end of second 1 and during second 4 in Figure 1.4. The positive phase reversals noted at the F8 derivation is due to the proximity of the cornea. The homologous F7 electrode site is negative due to the conjugate effect from the retina.

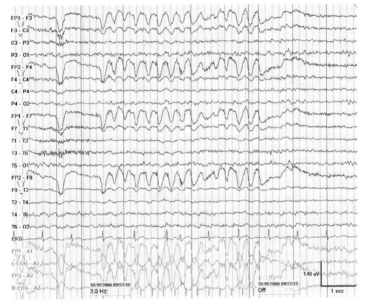

FIGURE 1.9. Eye movement monitors confirming a vertical eye flutter artifact with infraorbital electrodes (EOGs) during intermittent photic stimulation (IPS) to differentiate an artifact from frontal intermittent rhythmic delta activity (FIRDA).

Detecting eye movements may be accomplished using a single channel connecting the right upper lateral eyebrow and the left lower lateral eyebrow. However, because vertical eye movements are often the source of confusion, bilateral infraorbital electrodes referred to the ipsilateral ear as a reference may better represent the eye as a dipole and demonstrate phase reversals that are out-of-phase with cerebral activity when due to eye movements (see above). Eye movement monitors may be added during the recording if difficulty differentiating cerebral function from extracerebral origin becomes desirable.

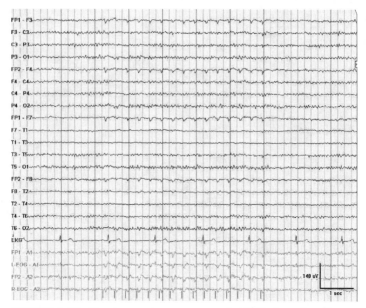

FIGURE 1.10. The electroretinogram seen at the FP1/2 electrodes <50 msec after the flash associated with intermittent photic stimulation.

The electroretinogram (ERG) is a normal response of the retina to photic stimulation. The amplitude is usually low voltage and appears in the anterior head regions. Normally an A and B wave are seen during evoked potential recording. However, the ERG can also be seen on the EEG and become confused with abnormal frontal sharp waves. To distinguish the ERG from the photoelectric effect, covering the electrodes with a clothe will demonstrate the persistence of the potentials. Additionally, high rates of IPS will fatigue the retinal response.

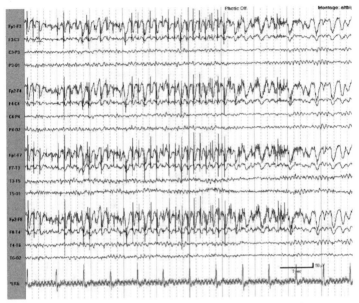

FIGURE 1.11. A photomyoclonic response during intermittent photic stimulation. Notice the spike-and-wave artifact created in the frontopolar channels.

The photomyoclonic response is an extracerebral response obtained from the frontalis muscles of the scalp. Contraction of the anterior muscles of the scalp produce EMG artifacts that vary from single to sustained myogenic potentials. The contractions are time locked to the photic stimulation and begin and cease commensurate with the flash, although there is often a brief delay between the flash and the myogenic potentials that appear. The principal confusion is one with a photoparoxysmal response (see above).

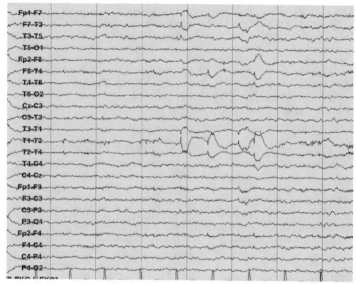

FIGURE 1.12. Prominent lateral rectus spikes during rapid eye movement (REM) sleep. Spikes occur with rapid eye movements to the left, right, left, and right in the 4th to 6th second.

Patients with rapid eye movements may demonstrate myogenic potentials from the lateral rectus muscles that may appear epileptiform in appearance. Each rapid eye movement is associated with a positive potential represented by a phase reversal on eye deviation to the side of the lateral rectus contracting.

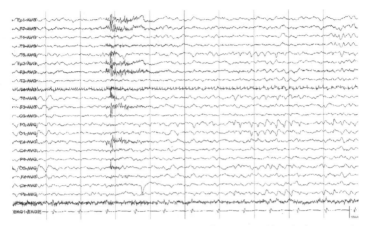

FIGURE 1.13. Muscle artifact at T4 manifests as repetitive single myogenic potentials. Oz has continuous single electrode artifact, and a bifrontal burst of muscle artifact is seen in second 3 to 4. Note the 6-Hz positive bursts in the 8th second. Filter settings are 1 to 70 Hz. (EEG courtesy of Greg Fisher MD).

Amyogenic (muscle) artifact consists of brief potentials that may occur individually or become continuous obscuring underlying EEG. EMG activity created during a seizure, during muscle contraction, or during movements are due to increased muscle tone. This artifact is most prominent in individuals who are tense during the EEG and is maximal in the temporal or frontopolar derivations (the site of frontalis musculature). Myogenic potentials are composed of high-frequency activity that is much briefer than the 20-msec potentials seen with epileptiform discharges. In addition, an aftergoing slow wave is absent, and having the individual relax their jaw muscles or capturing sleep will lead to waning or elimination of a myogenic artifact.

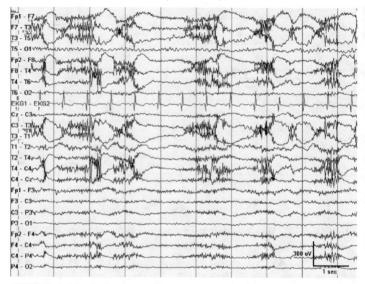

FIGURE 1.14. A chewing artifact seen at regular 1- to 2-second intervals. Note the continuous myogenic artifact in the bitemporal regions.

Regular bursts of myogenic potentials are seen during chewing. These high-voltage temporal predominant bursts are due to contraction of the muscles associated with mastication. Associated "slow" potentials during chewing reflect associated swallowing movements created by the tongue. The tongue, like the eye, acts as a dipole with the tip of the tongue being positive relative to the root. The chewing that is an effect created by the temporalis muscles is accompanied thereafter by the glossokinetic movements of the tongue.

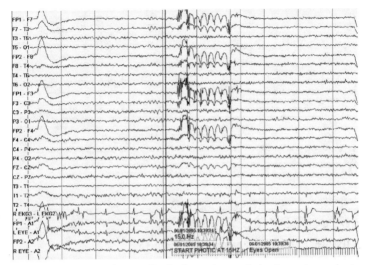

FIGURE 1.15. Pseudogeneralized spike-and-wave during intermittent photic stimulation due to superimposition of a physiological artifact from eye flutter and frontally predominant muscle artifact.

Superimposition of background frequencies can be deceiving when normal or artifactual frequencies are combined. Identifying normal morphologies within the background and comparing the frequencies of one or series of suspicious waveforms may help separate normal from abnormal. In the above example, combined artifacts (eye flutter and muscle artifact) create the appearance of a photoparoxysmal response during intermittent photic stimulation that could be a pitfall to novice interpreters.

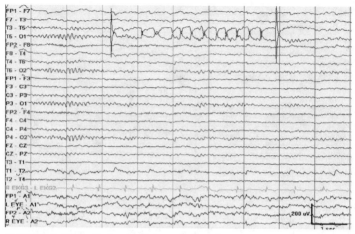

FIGURE 1.16A. Single electrode artifact at T5.

Potentials that are confined to a single electrode derivation are suspicious for a single (or common electrode in average/linked montages) electrode artifact. Identifying a single electrode artifact should prompt a technologist to check the impedance and resecure the electrode scalp-electrolyte interface, change the electrode with a persistent artifact, and/or move the electrode to an alternate channel to determine if the channel itself is defective.

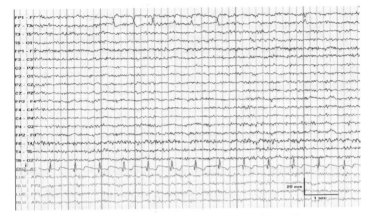

FIGURE 1.16B. Single electrode artifact at F7 mimicking a sharp wave.

Bizarre morphologies may occur and are usually recognizable. Occasionally a single electrode artifact may mimic sharp waves (see above).

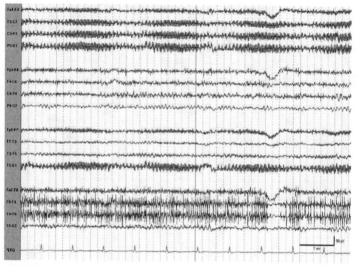

FIGURE 1.17A. A 60-Hz artifact.

A 60-cycle artifact is a function of the circuitry of the amplifiers and common mode rejection when electrode impedances are unequal. The frequency of an electrical line is represented in the EEG usually when poor electrode impedances produce a mismatch. This artifact should prompt a search for electrodes with an impedance of >5000 ohm when a single electrode is involved, as well as ensuring that ground loops and double grounds do not put the patient at a safety risk when generalized a 60-cycle artifact is found, as in the above example.

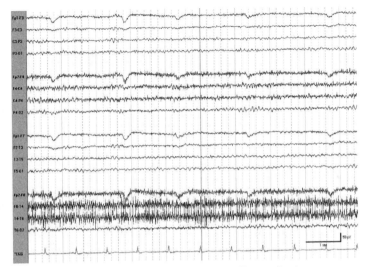

FIGURE 1.17B. A 60-Hz artifact after notched filter application.

After the application of the 60-Hz notched filter, note the elimination of the artifact that was seen on page 22 permitting interpretation of the unobscured EEG. However, notice the persistent right temporal myogenic artifact in the example above.

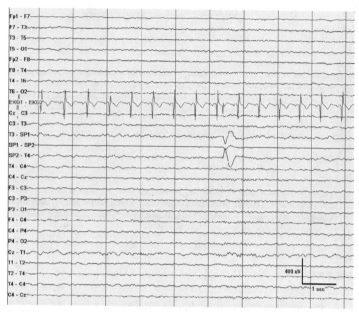

FIGURE 1.18. A sphenoidal artifact that appears as a temporal sharp wave. Note the absence of a lateral field in the left temporal chain.

Some electrode artifacts are difficult to recognize. In the above example, the sphenoidal derivations were not functional and created an electrode artifact that closely mimicked a temporal sharp wave. Note the lack of a believable cerebral field and the absence of any deflection in the true temporal and lateral temporal derivations despite the high amplitude reflected in the scale in the bottom right-hand corner.

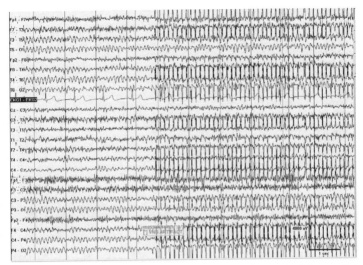

FIGURE 1.19. The vagus nerve stimulatior (VNS) artifact on the right recorded during stimulation while undergoing continuous video-EEG monitoring.

An electrical artifact occurs when electronic circuits surgically implanted (such as pacemakers or VNS) devices produce undesirable signals internally that contaminate the EEG or EKG recording. In this way, the patient or unshielded electrodes act as an antenna and produce extracerebral sources of artifact similar to the way nearby power lines may create external 60-Hz interference by the inducting magnetic fields created from nearby current flow. It is the current flow that results in electrode depolarization, is amplified by the amplifiers, and creates the resultant "noise."

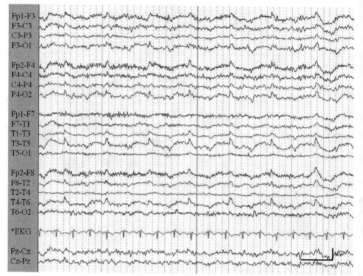

FIGURE 1.20. A mechanical artifact induced by CPAP in a comatose patient in the ICU. Note the alternating polarity of the mechanical artifact and low voltage.

A variety of artifacts can be see in the intensive care unit (ICU), critical care unit (CCU), or clinical specialty unit (CSU) produced by mechanical or instrumental sources. Electrical induced "noise" can be more evident for routine mechanical function at high gain (low sensitivity) settings. Alternating movement generated by a respirator is noted in the above example using high sensitivities of 3 µV/mm in a patient who is intubated and mechanically ventilated with continuous positive airway pressure (CPAP).

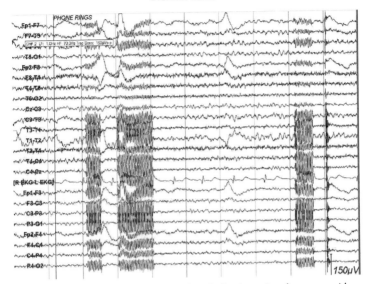

FIGURE 1.21. A telephone ring artifact during in-patient long-term video-EEG monitoring.

Environmental artifacts may be quite elusive. They may often not be readily identifiable or correctable within the confines of a "hostile" environment when performing EEG in the ICU or CCU. Some of these artifacts may be generated by high frequencies produced by nearby electrical machinery not directly connected to the patient. Equipment such as blood warmers, bovies, and electrical beds in the operating room (OR) may be challenging to locate the source of the artifact. By unplugging or moving equipment away from the recording electrode, redirecting electrical current flow may eliminate the artifact from the EEG. Telephone lines (see above) may interfere with EEG and produce an artifact typically in all the channels during recording.

NORMAL EEG

The application of routine EEG provides information about generators emanating from a three-dimensional sphere with regard to location, distribution, waveform frequency, polarity, and morphology. The state of wakefulness and age are critical features for accurate interpretation of the normal EEG.

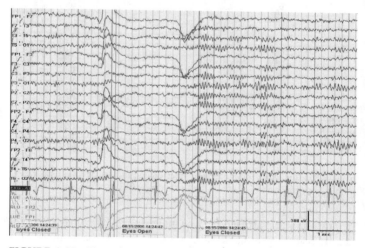

FIGURE 1.22. Normal 10-Hz alpha rhythm "blocked" by eye opening and returning on eye closure. Note the faster frequency immediately on eye closure ("squeak").

The alpha rhythm remains the starting point to analyze clinical EEG. In the normal EEG, a posterior dominant rhythm is represented bilaterally over the posterior head regions and lies within the 8- to 13-Hz bandwidth (*alpha frequency*). When this rhythm is attenuated with eye opening, it is referred to as the *alpha rhythm*. During normal development, an 8-Hz alpha frequency appears by 3 years of age. The alpha rhythm remains stable between 8 and 12 Hz even during normal aging into the later years of life. In approximately one-fourth of normal adults, the alpha rhythm is poorly visualized, and in

<10%, voltages of <15 µV may be seen. The alpha rhythm is distributed maximally in the occipital regions, and shifts anteriorly during drowsiness. Voltage asymmetries of >50% should be regarded as being abnormal, especially when the left side is greater than the right. It is best observed during relaxed wakefulness, and has a side to side difference of <1 Hz. Unilateral failure of the alpha rhythm to attenuate reflects an ipsilateral abnormality (*Bancaud's phenomenon*). Normally, alpha frequencies may transiently increase immediately after eye closure (*alpha squeak*). Alpha variants include forms that are one-half (slow alpha) or two times (fast alpha) the frequency with similar distribution and reactivity. Alpha variants may have a notched appearance. *Paradoxical alpha* occurs when alertness results in the presence of alpha, and drowsiness does not.

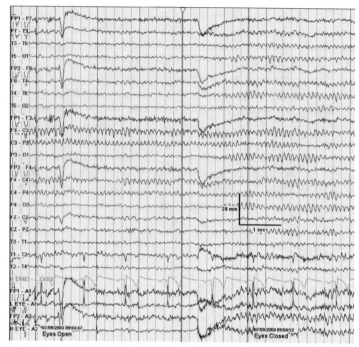

FIGURE 1.23. Note the prominent left central mu rhythm during eye opening.

The mu rhythm is a centrally located arciform alpha frequency (usually 8 to 10 Hz) that represents the sensorimotor cortex at rest (Figure 1.23). While it resembles the alpha rhythm, it does not block with eye opening, but instead with contralateral movement of an extremity. It may be seen only on one side, and may be quite asymmetrical and asynchronous, despite the notable absence of an underlying structural lesion. The mu rhythm may slow with advancing age, and is usually of lower amplitude than the existent alpha rhythm. When persistent, unreactive, and associated with focal slowing, mulike frequencies are abnormal.

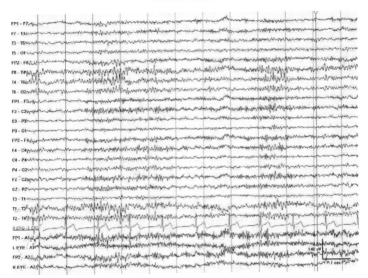

FIGURE 1.24. Breach rhythm in the right temporal region (maximal at T4) following craniotomy for temporal lobectomy.

Beta rhythms are frequencies that are more than 13 Hz. They are common, and normally observed within the 18- to 25-Hz bandwidth with a voltage of <20 μV. Voltages beyond 25 μV in amplitude are abnormal. Benzodiazepines, barbiturates, and chloral hydrate are potent generalized beta activators of "fast activity" >50 μV for >50% of the waking tracing within the 14- to 16-Hz bandwidth. Beta activity normally increases during drowsiness, light sleep, and with mental activation. Persistently reduced voltages of >50% suggest a cortical gray matter abnormality within the hemisphere having the lower amplitude; however, lesser asymmetries may simply reflect normal skull asymmetries. A skull defect may produce a *breach rhythm* with focal, asymmetrical, higher amplitudes (this relative increase may be more than three times) beta activity without the skull to attenuate the faster frequencies. It is normal unless associated with spikes or focal slowing.

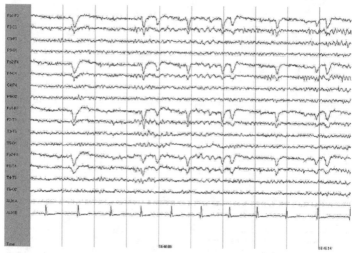

FIGURE 1.25. Normal frontocentral theta rhythm in an 18-year-old patient while awake.

Theta rhythms are composed of 4- to 7-Hz frequencies of varying amplitude and morphologies. Approximately one-third of normal awake, young adults show intermittent 6- to 7-Hz theta rhythms of <15 μV that is maximal in the frontal or frontocentral head regions. The appearance of frontal theta can be facilitated by emotions, focused concentration, and during mental tasks. Theta activity is normally enhanced by hyperventilation, drowsiness, and sleep. Intermittent 4- to 5-Hz activity bitemporally, or even with a lateralized predominance (usually left > right), may occur in about one-third of the asymptomatic elderly and is not abnormal.

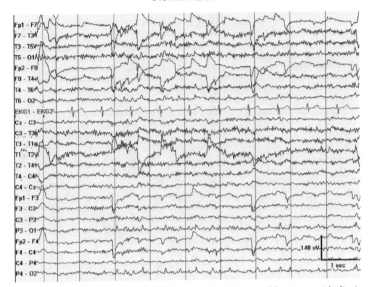

FIGURE 1.26. Biooccipital lambda waves in a 28-year-old patient with dizziness. Notice the frequent "scanning" eye movement artifact in the F7 and T8 derivations.

Lambda waves have been initially described as surface positive sharply contoured theta waves appearing bilaterally in the occipital region. These potentials have a duration of 160 to 250 msec, and may at times be quite sharply contoured, asymmetrical, with higher amplitudes than the resting posterior dominant rhythm. When they occur asymmetrically, they may be confusion with interictal epileptiform discharges, and potentially lead to the misinterpretation of the EEG. They are best observed in young adults when seen, although they are more frequently found in children. Lambda waves are best elicited when the patient visually scans a textured or complex picture with fast saccadic eye movements. Placing a white sheet of paper in front of the individual will eliminate the visual input that is essential for their genesis.

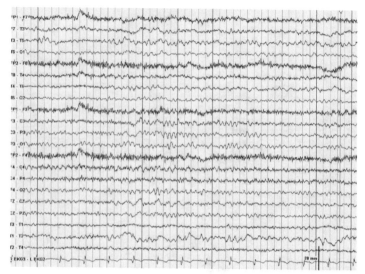

FIGURE 1.27. Intermittent left mid-temporal delta during transition to drowsiness in a normal 84-year-old patient evaluated for syncope.

Delta rhythms are frequencies consist of <4-Hz activity that comprises <10% of the normal waking EEG by age 10 years. In the waking states, delta can be considered a normal finding in the very young and in the elderly. The normal elderly may have rare irregular delta complexes in the temporal regions. It is similar to temporal theta in the distribution, often left > right temporal head regions, but normally is present for <1% of the recording. Some delta is normal in people older than 60 years, at the onset of drowsiness, in response to hyperventilation, and during slow-wave sleep. Excessive generalized delta is abnormal and indicates an encephalopathy that is etiology nonspecific. Focal arrhythmic delta usually indicates a structural lesion involving the white matter of the ipsilateral hemisphere, especially when it is continuous and unreactive.

NORMAL SLEEP ARCHITECTURE

Stage 1 sleep is defined by the presence of vertex waves, typically 200-msec diphasic sharp transients with maximal negativity at the vertex (Cz) electrode. They may be seen in stages 1 to 3 sleep. They are bilateral, synchronous, and symmetrical, and may be induced by auditory stimuli. Vertex waves can appear spiky (especially in children) but should normally never be consistently lateralized. Other features include attenuation of the alpha rhythm, greater frontal prominence of beta, slow rolling eye movements, and vertex sharp transients. In addition, positive occipital sharp transients (POSTS) are another feature signifying stage 1 sleep. These are surface positive, bisynchronous physiological sharp waves with voltage asymmetries that may occur over the occipital regions as single complexes or in repetitive bursts that may be present in both stages 1 and 2 sleep.

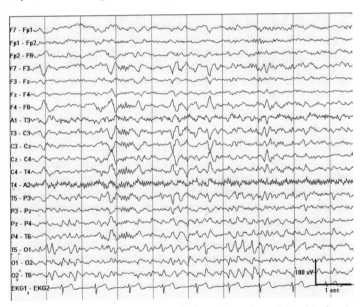

FIGURE 1.28. POSTS appearing in the lower three channels in a bipolar circle montage demonstrating positive polarity in the occipital region during sleep. Notice the surface negative vertex waves maximal at Cz.

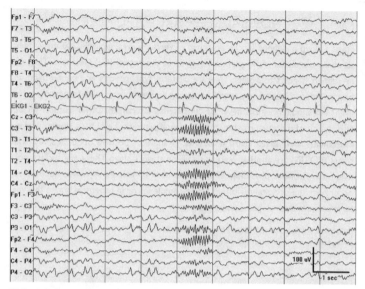

FIGURE 1.29. Stage 2 sleep with prominent sleep spindles and POSTs.

Stage 2 sleep is defined by the presence of sleep spindles and K complexes. This stage has the same features as stage 1 with progressive slowing of background frequencies. Sleep spindles are transient, sinusoidal 12- to 14-Hz activity with waxing and waning amplitude seen in the central regions with frontal representation by slower frequencies of 10 to 12 Hz. A *K-complex* is a high amplitude diphasic wave with an initial sharp transient followed by a high-amplitude slow wave often associated with a sleep spindle in the frontocentral regions. A K-complex may be evoked by a sudden auditory stimulus. A persistent asymmetry of >50% is abnormal on the side of reduction.

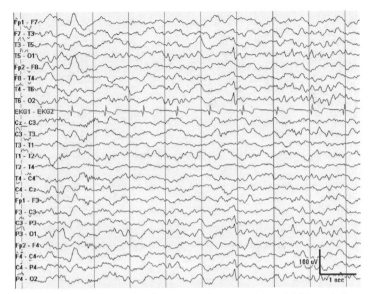

FIGURE 1.30. Slow-wave sleep. Note the intermittent POSTs and sleep spindles against the continuous delta background.

Slow-wave sleep now best describes non-REM deep sleep and is comprised of 1- to 2-Hz delta frequencies occupying variable amounts of the background. Stage 3 previously noted delta occupying 20% to 50% of the recording with voltages of >75 μV, while stage 4 consists of delta present for >50% of the recording.

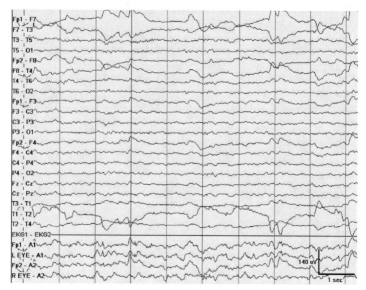

FIGURE 1.31. REM sleep with rapid eye movements associated with lateral rectus spikes is noted at the F7 and F8 derivations.

REM sleep is characterized by rapid eye movements, loss of muscle tone, and saw-toothed waves in the EEG (Figure 1.10). Non-REM and REM sleep alternate in cycles four to six times during a normal night's sleep. A predominance of non-REM appears in the first part of the night, and REM in the last third of the night. A routine EEG with REM may reflect sleep deprivation and not necessarily a disorder of sleep-onset REM such as narcolepsy.

ACTIVATION PROCEDURES

Activation techniques are a useful part of EEG in clinical practice and represent various types of stimuli or modalities that are able to trigger abnormalities. Hyperventilation and intermittent photic stimulation are routinely performed to augment slowing and/or epileptiform abnormalities, although sleep deprivation, pharmacological, and other methods may be employed.

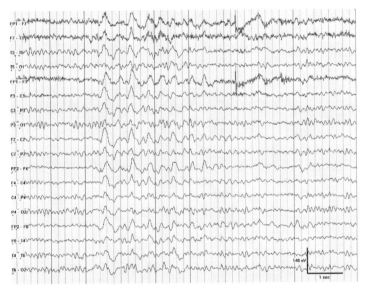

FIGURE 1.32. Normal build-up during hyperventilation.

Hyperventilation is routinely performed for 3 to 5 minutes in most EEG laboratories. The purpose is to create cerebral vasoconstriction through respiratory means promoting systemic hypocarbia. Hyperventilation normally produces a bilateral increase in theta and delta frequencies (build-up) that is frontally predominant, and often of high amplitude. Resolution of the effect occurs normally within 1 minute. Activation, or the generation of epileptiform discharges, is infrequently seen in those with localization-related epilepsy (<10%);

however, this may approach 80% for those with generalized epilepsies that include absence seizures. Hyperventilation may produce focal slowing in patients with an underlying structural lesion. It should not be performed in patients with severe cardiac or pulmonary disease, acute or recent stroke, significant large vessel cerebrovascular, and sickle cell anemia or trait, and it should be used with caution during pregnancy.

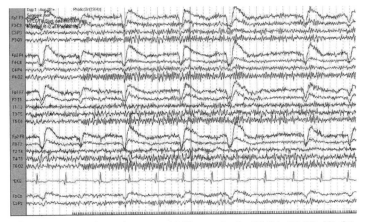

FIGURE 1.33. Photic driving at 20 Hz seen in the P3-O1, P4-O2, T5-O1, and T6-O2 derivations.

Intermittent photic stimulation normally produces potentials exquisitely time locked to the frequency of the intermittent light stimulus, and is referred to as *photic driving*. Response depends upon background illumination and the distance of the light source from the patient. Distances of <30 cm from the patient are used to optimize the effect of stimulation. Flashes are very brief, and delivered in sequence from 1 to 30 Hz flash frequencies for approximately 10 sec before stopping the stimulus. Subharmonics and harmonics of the flash frequency may be seen. Photic driving is usually greatest in the occipital location, in frequencies approximating the alpha rhythm, when the eyes are closed. *Photomyoclonic* (or *photomyogenic*) *responses* consist of a frontally dominant muscle artifact that occurs when the flash evokes repetitive local contraction of the frontalis musculature (photomyogenic). The periocular muscles may also be affected with single lightening-like head jerks (photomyoclonic). Myogenic spikes occur 50 to 60 msec after the flash and increase in amplitude as the stimulus frequency increases. The response is normal, although it may be seen is withdrawal syndromes or states of hyperexcitability.

41

BENIGN VARIANTS OF UNCERTAIN SIGNIFICANCE

Patterns that are rhythmic or epileptiform are often features that are associated with an abnormal EEG. Known patterns of uncertain significance or "benign variants" may possess these same characteristics and may reflect pitfalls for those interpreting EEG.

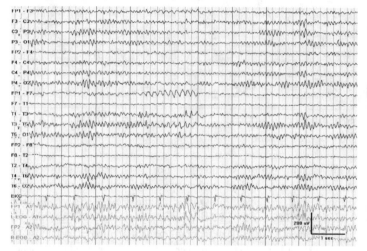

FIGURE 1.34. Rhythmic temporal theta bursts of drowsiness. Note the sharply contoured morphology.

Rhythmic temporal theta bursts of drowsiness is now the preferred term for what was previously described as a psychomotor variant. This pattern occurs in 0.5% to 2.0% of selected normal adults and consists of bursts or runs of 5- to 7-Hz theta waves that may appear sharp, flat, or notched in appearance. It is maximal in the midtemporal derivations and was referred to as rhythmic mid-temporal theta bursts of drowsiness. It is an interictal pattern that does not evolve spatially or temporally, although it may be represented bilaterally or independently over both hemispheres. It is seen in adolescents and adults in relaxed wakefulness.

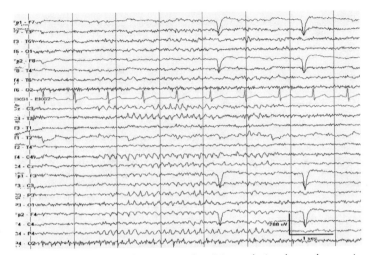

FIGURE 1.35. Central theta (maximal at Cz) seen during the awake state in a 35-year-old patient with migraine headaches.

A focal sinusoidal or arciform 4- to 7-Hz theta rhythm maximally expressed over the midline vertex region was first described by Ciganek. While morphologically it may resemble a mu rhythm, it is not similarly reactive, and is slower in frequency, and occurs both in drowsiness or the alert state. While initially felt to be a projected rhythm in temporal lobe epilepsy, it has been seen in a heterogeneous population and is therefore of nonspecific clinical significance.

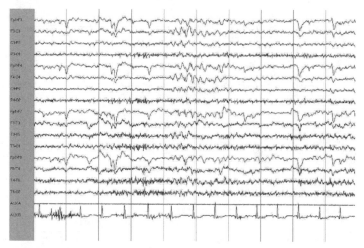

FIGURE 1.36. A 6-Hz (phantom) spike-wave burst with frontal predominance in the 5th second of this EEG in an awake patient with temporal lobe epilepsy.

Spike-and-wave discharges at 6 Hz were first known as "phantom spike-and-waves." The acronyms WHAM (wakefulness, high amplitude, anterior, male) and FOLD (female, occipital, low amplitude, drowsy) were used to describe the two primary subtypes. Bilateral, synchronous, 6-Hz spike-and-wave discharges may range from 5 to 7 Hz, although with a typical repetition rate of 6 Hz lasting briefly for 1 to 2 sec. The spike is often of very low amplitude, at times difficult to appreciate during routine interpretation of the EEG by qualitative visual analysis. When the spikes are of low amplitude and occur only during drowsiness, they usually represent benign finding. When they are seen with high-amplitude spikes and occur with less than a 6-Hz frequency, or occur during wakefulness and persist into slow-wave sleep, there is a greater association with seizures.

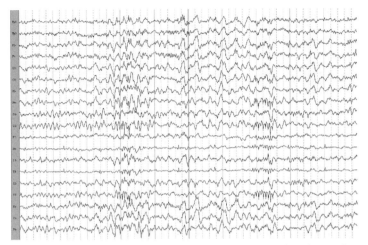

FIGURE 1.37. Fourteen- and 6-Hz positive bursts maximal in the T6 electrode derivation in a linked-ears reference montage. Note the downward deflection and prominent 14-Hz frequency.

Fourteen- and 6-Hz positive bursts (originally called 14 and 6-Hz positive spikes) have also been called ctenoids. They appear in the EEG in bursts of positive comb-like spindles mainly over the posterior temporal head regions. They are present most frequently at a rate of 14 or 6 to 7 Hz and last 0.5 to 1.0 sec in duration. The 14-Hz frequency is most prevalent, and the 6- Hz burst may appear with or without the faster frequencies. They are most common during adolescence, although they may persist into adulthood and decrease with age. The bursts are usually unilateral or bilaterally asynchronous with a shifting predominance involving one hemisphere to a greater degree. A contralateral ear reference montage and greater interelectrode distance best demonstrate these bursts.

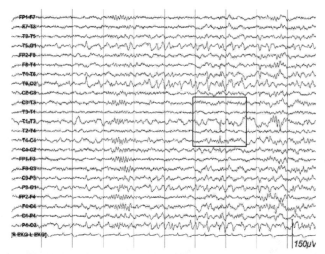

FIGURE 1.38. A right benign epileptiform transients of sleep (BETS) in the temporal region during stage 2 sleep. Note the higher amplitude in the T1 and T2 channel with a longer interelectrode distance.

Different terms describe the small sharp spikes. or benign epileptiform transients of sleep, or benign sporadic sleep spikes of sleep that depict a low-voltage (<50 μV), brief-duration (<50 msec), simple waveform with a monophasic or diphasic spike. This benign variant of uncertain significance has the morphology of a spike, although it has an rapidly ascending limb and steep descending limb best seen in the anterior to mid-temporal derivations during non-REM sleep. They are most common in adults. They may be >50 μV, have a duration >50 msec, and may appear with an aftergoing slow-wave (usually of lower amplitude than the spike). They are not associated with focal slowing. They do not occur in runs. The most distinguishing characteristic is that they disappear in slow-wave sleep. They appear as a unilateral discharge but are almost always independent when they are bilateral. They may possess a field that may correspond to an oblique transverse dipole resulting in opposite polarities over opposite hemispheres when they are bilateral.

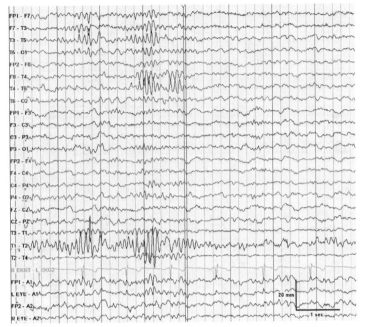

FIGURE 1.39. Wicket waves maximal at T3 and T4.

Wicket spikes are most commonly seen in adults >30 years of age. They occur within the 6- to 11-Hz band, and can obtain amplitudes of up to 200 µV. They are seen over the temporal regions during drowsiness and light sleep and are usually bilateral and independent. They typically occur in bursts, although they may be confused with interictal epileptiform discharges, especially when they occur independently or as isolated waveforms. No focal slowing or aftergoing slow-wave component is seen, and they likely represent fragmented temporal alpha activity. Similar frequency and morphology of bursts to the isolated waveforms is a means of providing support for the nonepileptogenic origin. Wicket waves are considered an epileptiform normal variant though they may be easily mistaken as abnormal sharp waves.

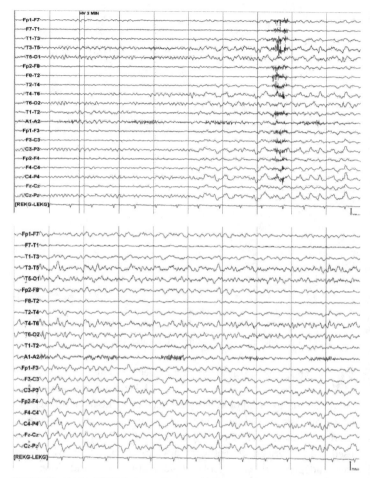

FIGURE 1.40. SREDA in a 73-year-old patient during hyperventilation (HV). No clinical signs were present.

In contrast to many of the patterns of uncertain significance that mimic IEDs, subclinical rhythmic electrographic discharge in adults (SREDA) is a pattern that mimics the epileptiform characteristics of a subclinical seizure. However, no clinical features exist during it, either subjective or objective findings, and no association with epilepsy has been demonstrated. In contrast to most benign variants, SREDA is more likely to occur in those over 50 years of age and also while the person is awake. It may exist in two forms, either as a bilateral episodic burst of rhythmic sharply contoured 5- to 7-Hz theta frequencies appearing maximal over the temporoparietal derivations or as an abrupt mononphasic series of repetitive sharp or slow waveforms that appear focally at the vertex recurring in progressively shorter intervals until a sustained burst is noted. Rarely the two forms may appear in the same person (personal observation WOT). Bursts of SREDA usually last between 40 and 80 sec and occur without postictal slowing.

CHAPTER 1

ADDITIONAL RESOURCES

Abou-Knalil B, Misulis KE. *Atlas of EEG and Seizure Semiology*. Butterworth Heinemann, Philadelphia, 2006:1–213.

Benbadis SR, Tatum WO. Overinterpretation of EEGs and misdiagnosis of epilepsy. *J Clin Neurophysiol* 2003;20:42–44.

Blume WT, Masako K, Young GB. Atlas of Adult *Electroencephalography*. 2nd ed. Lippincott Williams & Wilkins, Philadelphia, 2002:1–531.

Kellaway Peter. Orderly approach to visual analysis: elements of the normal EEG and their characteristics in children and adults. In: Ebersole JS, Pedley TA, eds. *Current Practice of Clinical Electroencephalography*. 3rd ed. Lippincott Williams & Wilkins, Philadelphia, 2003:100–159.

Markand, Omkar N. Pearls, perils, and pitfalls in the use of the electroencephalogram. *Semin Neurol* 2003;23(1):7–46.

Olejniczak P. Neurophysiologic basis of EEG. *J Clin Neurophysiol* 2006;23(3): 186–189.

Tatum WO, IV, Husain A, Benbadis SR, Kaplan PW. Normal human adult EEG and normal variants. *J Clin Neurophysiol* 2006;23(3):194–207.

Westmoreland BF. Benign electroencephalographic variants and patterns of uncertain clinical significance. In: Ebersole JS, Pedley TA, eds. *Current Practice of Clinical Electroencephalography*. 3rd ed. Lippincott Williams & Wilkins, Philadelphia, 2003:235–245.

Abnormal Nonepileptiform EEG

SELIM R. BENBADIS

Interictal EEG provides information about the presence of nonepileptiform electrophysiological dysfunction. When abnormalities are encountered, they are not specific for an underlying etiology, and as such represent abnormalities without further differentiation of the pathological process. While neuroimaging demonstrates anatomical definition, EEG provides evidence of organic electrophysiological dysfunction.

The EEG is sensitive to cerebral dysfunction, but may have a lag during clinical improvement or lead relative to maximal clinical symptomatology. Many of the patterns that are nonepileptiform are nonspecific in etiology, yet the presence of abnormality is often a reflection of the clinical presence and degree of dysfunction. Acuity is unable to be demonstrated by EEG in nonepileptiform abnormalities, although serial tracing may further help to define the trend toward neurological evolution of improvement or deterioration. Therefore, EEG is able objectively to substantiate and quantify to a degree the depth of encephalopathy when diffuse nonepileptiform abnormalities are encountered and lateralize (or even localize) abnormalities when focal areas of slowing are evident. Many nonepileptiform and epileptiform abnormalities characterize encephalopathy. This chapter will

51

focus on generalized and focal nonepileptiform abnormalities. Chapters 3 and 5 will discuss patterns that are associated with epileptiform abnormalities and patterns of special significance.

DIFFUSE SLOWING

Diffuse slowing on the EEG may have various morphologies, and occur intermittently or continuously, to reflect abnormal cerebral function. The presence of diffuse slowing suggests a bilateral disturbance of cerebral function and represents an encephalopathy that is nonspecific for etiology.

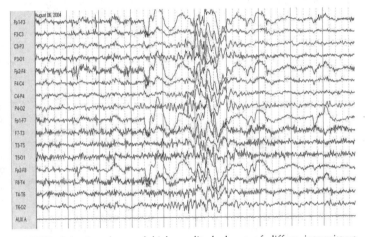

FIGURE 2.1. An abnormal high-amplitude burst of diffuse intermittent theta in an awake adult following a motor vehicle accident associated with driving under the influence.

Intermixed diffuse intermittent theta in the most alert state is normal in young adults. When theta frequencies are seen in the frontal or frontocentral regions and voltages are >100 µV or when theta is present >10% of the time in an adult (not in childhood or elderly), then theta may reflect a nonspecific abnormality similar to diffuse intermittent slowing or background slowing, but may be seen normally in young adults. The slower the frequency, the higher the amplitude, and the greater the persistence, the more likely intermittent theta is abnormal.

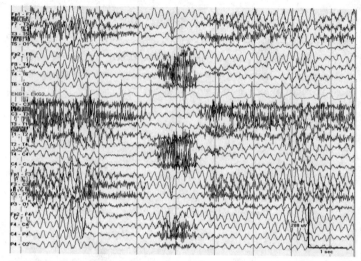

FIGURE 2.2. Generalized monomorphic 5 to 6-Hz theta frequencies obtained during syncope in a patient undergoing head-up tilt table testing for neurocardiogenic syncope.

Diffuse (or generalized) slowing in the background reflects a nonspecific abnormality and is indicative of a bilateral disturbance of cerebral function. Progression of abnormal intermixed intermittent slowing in the case of generalized abnormal nonepileptiform features include initially intermixed intermittent theta (sometimes normal as discussed above), with a greater degree of abnormality, intermittent slowing becomes continous and theta slowing is replaced by delta frequencies.

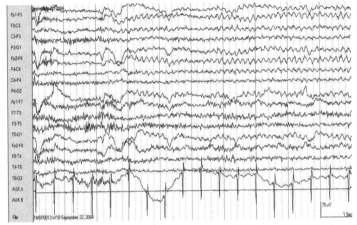

FIGURE 2.3. Slowing of the posterior dominant rhythm to 6 Hz. This well-defined background is too slow even in a 65-year-old man.

Background slowing is defined as slowing of the normal posterior background activity to a frequency slower than the normal alpha rhythm frequency of <8 Hz and is an early finding of encephalopathy. The degree of slowing of the background reflects the degree of cerebral dysfunction. This pattern is defined as a posterior dominant rhythm that is present and normally reactive, but too slow for age. The lower limits of normal for the alpha rhythm is 5, 6, 7, and 8 Hz at ages 1, 3, 5, and 8 years old, respectively. Often times, diffuse slowing of the background is associated with other stigmata of mild diffuse encephalopathy such as intermittent bursts of generalized theta or delta activity.

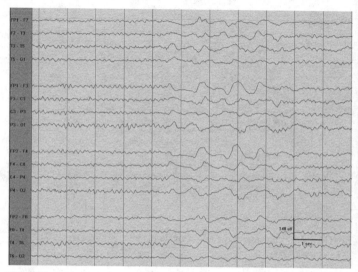

FIGURE 2.4. An intermittent 4-sec burst of 1- to 2-Hz irregular delta activity. This 55-year- old woman was clinically confused and disoriented, with multiple metabolic and systemic disturbances.

Diffuse intermittent slowing is characterized by intermittent bursts of diffuse slow activity, usually in the delta range, that appear often in excess of the background slowing (see above). Like background slowing, with which it frequently coexists, it is indicative of a mild diffuse encephalopathy. The bursts are usually polymorphic but can occasionally be rhythmic. As the severity of the encephalopathy increases, the bursts will increase in duration and frequency and merge into or become continuous generalized slowing (see continuous generalized slowing, page 59). Like other encephalopathic patterns, this is nonspecific as to etiology. Diffuse intermittent slowing may reflect either a cortical or subcortical cerebral dysfunction.

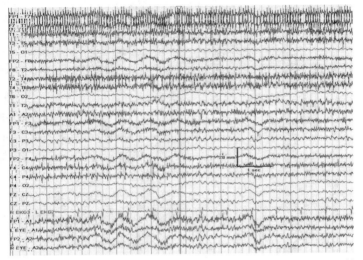

FIGURE 2.5. Frontal intermittent rhythmic delta activity in a 67-year-old patient with noncommunicating hydrocephalus. Note the slower 1.0- to 1.5-Hz frequency and cerebral origin verified by eye monitors.

Frontal intermittent rhythmic delta activity (FIRDA) appears in bursts of delta that is often high voltage, bisynchronous, and well formed. FIRDA may rarely be asymmetrical. This abnormal pattern when seen in the waking adult EEG consists of bilateral rhythmic monomorphic delta waves with a consistent frequency throughout the EEG. Bifrontal predominance is typical in adults, and occipital predominance is more typically seen in children, changing with brain maturation. FIRDA is most often associated with encephalopathies of toxic or metabolic origin, although it may also occur with subcortical lesions such as a deep midline lesion or increased intracranial pressure.

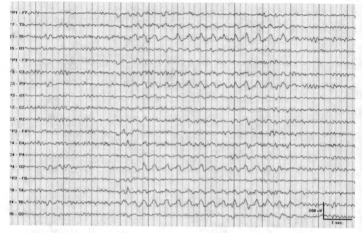

FIGURE 2.6. ORIDA in a 6-year-old child with absence epilepsy.

Occipital intermittent rhythmic delta activity (OIRDA), like FIRDA, is a nonspecific finding in the EEG relative to etiology. OIRDA is demonstrated as a posterior predominant bisynchronous rhythmic delta slowing appearing in bursts. OIRDA has the same features as FIRDA but occurs in children. OIRDA appears maximal over the occipital region instead of appearing with frontal predominance. OIRDA has been noted to occur in association with generalized (absence) epilepsy, but is not an epileptiform abnormality unless intermixed spikes are present.

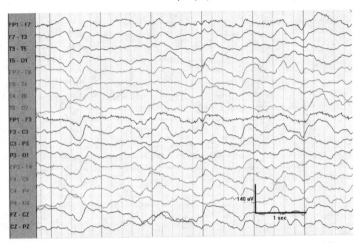

FIGURE 2.7. Continuous irregular 1.5- to 3.0-Hz delta in a 66-year-old man with encephalopathy that was unresponsive. The above example of EEG is representative of the entire record. No reactivity was noted during the EEG.

Continuous generalized slowing consists of polymorphic delta activity that is continuous or near-continuous (>80% of the record) and (at least as importantly) unreactive. *Unreactive* implies no change with external stimuli and also the absence of sleep-wake patterns. Unlike the prior two patterns (background slowing and intermittent generalized slowing), this pattern is indicative of a severe diffuse encephalopathy, and most patients with this pattern are comatose or nearly so. Like other encephalopathic patterns, this is nonspecific as to etiology. The most common causes by far are metabolic or systemic disturbances, although severe diffuse lesions affecting the brain can also produce this pattern (e.g., traumatic brain injuries or advanced neurodegenerative diseases).

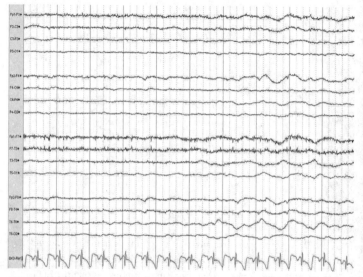

FIGURE 2.8. Low-voltage recording in a patient involved in a motor vehicle accident. The recording was obtained at a sensitivity of 2 μV/mm with no voltage of >20 μV.

Low-voltage EEG is typically associated with diffuse slowing of the background rhythm. In general, the state of the patient is the best indicator of abnormality with some low-voltage EEGs of <10 to 20 μV found in a subset of normal individuals. When seen during encephalopathy or coma, low-voltage EEG is typically associated with diffuse slowing and poor reactivity to somatosensory stimulation. One distinguishing characteristic is the lack of admixed alpha and beta frequencies in this low-voltage recording.

FOCAL ABNORMALITIES

Focal abnormalities on the EEG provide electrographic evidence of a localized abnormal cerebral function. They are not specific for etiology and may be seen with many different underlying structural lesions that affect the brain. They may also be encountered as a temporary non-structural physiological effect (i.e., following a seizure). The location, morphology, persistence, and poor reactivity are features that suggest an underlying structural lesion, but because the specificity is low, a broad differential is required.

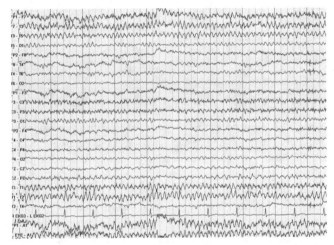

FIGURE 2.9. Alpha asymmetry in a patient with an acute right frontoparietal ischemic infarction.

Alpha asymmetries depict an abnormality on the side ipsilateral to the hemisphere and characteristically involve a slow posterior dominant rhythm. Additional focal, regional, or lateralized abnormalities are often seen in conjunction with alpha asymmetries. A persistent hemispheric difference of >1 Hz should be regarded as being abnormal when alpha asymmetry is seen. Additionally, while the right hemisphere is often asymmetrical in respect to voltage, a persistent amplitude asymmetry of >50% should be regarded as abnormal.

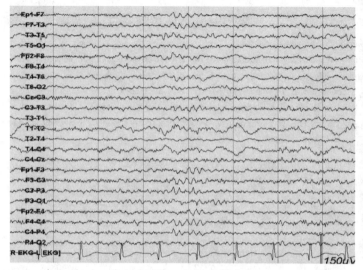

FIGURE 2.10. Focal delta in a 28-year-old patient with right temporal polymorphic delta due to a anterior temporal ganglioglioma. Note the anterior–mid-temporal localization with loss of intermixed faster frequencies.

Focal polymorphic delta is confined to one to two electrode contacts and indicates a more restricted disturbance of cerebral dysfunction affecting the white matter tracts. When concomitant loss of faster frequencies is seen (above), EEG may be more suggestive of a structural lesion, but may also be seen with any structural lesion that affects both grey and white matter.

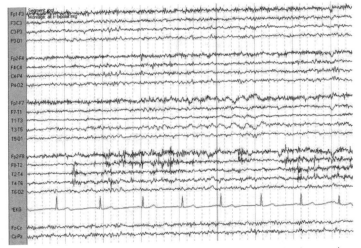

FIGURE 2.11. Temporal intermittent rhythmic delta activity in a patient with left temporal lobe epilepsy.

Temporal intermittent rhythmic delta activity (TIRDA) is a unique form of intermittent rhythmic delta activity. It consists of an intermittent monomorphic burst of delta frequencies maximal typically in a unilateral temporal derivation. The presence of TIRDA has a strong association with partial seizures. It may provide localizing capabilities in patients with temporal lobe epilepsy. TIRDA is often associated with interictal epileptiform discharges (IEDs) and is abnormal.

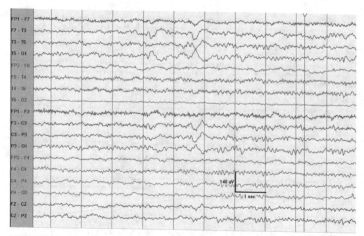

FIGURE 2.12. There is a brief 2-sec burst of polymorphic delta activity in the posterior temporal-parietal region of the left hemisphere in a 55-year-old patient with a left subcortical white matter lacunar infarction.

Intermittent slowing has a low correlation with an underlying lesion compared to focal slowing that is continuous. Focal slowing may indicate an underlying structural lesion involving the white matter tracts of the brain. Definite statements about the etiology of the slowing activity cannot be made by appearance on the EEG.

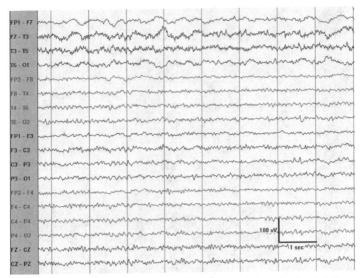

FIGURE 2.13. A 75-year-old patient with an acute left frontal ischemic infarct. Note the left regional polymorphic delta that affects the entire hemisphere.

Continuous regional delta slowing on the EEG has a high correlation with an underlying structural lesion involving the white matter of the ipsilateral hemisphere. The area of slowing usually overlies the hemisphere containing the structural lesion, but does not necessarily reflect the exact location as the one represented by EEG. Trauma, tumor, stroke, intracranial hemorrhages, and infection appear similar on the EEG without specific features.

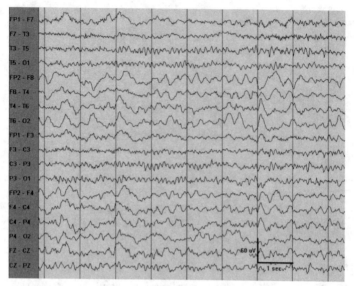

FIGURE 2.14. A 64-year-old s/p right hemisphere infarct. Over the right hemisphere, a well-formed alpha rhythm is not present (it is well formed on the left) and is replaced by polymorphic slow waves (2 to 4 Hz).

Lateralized polymorphic delta slowing may consist of theta or delta frequencies that are focal, regional, or lateralized. Delta that is polymorphic (or arrhythmic) is composed of slow-wave activity that is 3.5 Hz (or less) and is composed of waveforms that vary in frequency and duration. Polymorphic delta activity when localized is indicative of an underlying supratentorial lesion affecting the white matter of the ipsilateral hemisphere. The greater the state-independence and persistence, the greater the degree of correlation with a structural lesion. Localized polymorphic delta, however, may be seen as a transitory phenomenon from head injury, transient ischemic attack, migraine, and during a postictal state.

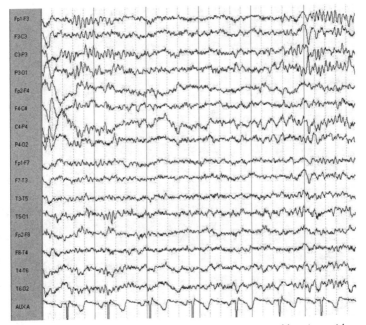

FIGURE 2.15. Asymmetry of sleep spindles in a 36-year-old patient with a right thalamic glioma.

Sleep spindles are initially evident in the first 2 months, and by 2 years of age are synchronous in normal children. Sleep elements are normally maximal in frequency in the central location, although they may appear in the frontal regions as well. A frequency of 12 to 14 Hz is observed in the central regions and is the distinguishing characteristic of stage 2 sleep. Spindles are very stable in the bilateral appearance, and a persistent slowing of frequency or unilateral appearance should be regarded as an abnormal nonepileptiform feature.

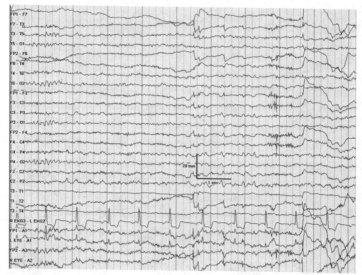

FIGURE 2.16. Sleep-onset REM in a 39-year-old patient with narcolepsy.

Sleep-onset rapid eye movement (REM) is extremely rare in normal individuals. The effect of sleep deprivation and sedative medication are exceptions that may be seen to create this phenomenon in the EEG laboratory if the EEG is obtained closely approximating sleep. For most, disorders of excessive daytime sleepiness are associated with sleep-onset REM and narcolepsy has been the principal (though not exclusive) sleep disorder that it denotes. Ensuring a night of adequate sleep before demonstrating at least two naps with sleep-onset REM is found in the context of the clinical history of excessive daytime sleepiness.

ADDITIONAL RESOURCES

Benbadis SR. Focal disturbances of brain function. In: Levin KH, Lüders HO, eds. *Comprehensive Clinical Neurophysiology.* Philadelphia, Saunders, 2000:457–467.

Epstein CM, Riecher AM, Henderson RM, et al. EEG in liver transplantatioin: visual and comnputerized analysis. *Electroencephalogr Clin Neurophysiol* 1992;83:367–371.

Gloor P, Kalabay O, Giard N. The electroencephalogram in diffuse encephalopathies: electroenephalographic correlates of grey and white matter lesions. *Brain* 1968;91:779–802.

Kaplan PW. Metabolic and endocrine disorders resenbling seizures. In: Engel J Jr, Pedley TA, eds. *Epilepsy: A Comprehensive Textbook.* Philadelphia: Lippincott Raven, 1997:2661–2670.

Liporace J, Tatum W, Morris GL, et al. Clinical utility of sleep-deprived versus computer-assisted ambulatory 16-channel EEG in epilepsy patients: a multi-center study. *Epilep Res* 1998;32:357–362.

Luders H, Noachtar S, eds. *Atlas and Classification of Electroencephalography.* Philadelphia, Saunders, 2000.

Schaul N, Gloor P, Gotman J. The EEG in deep midline lesions. *Neurology* 1981;31:157-167.

Zifkin BG, Cracco RQ. An orderly approach to the abnormal electroencephalogram. In: Ebersole JS, Pedley TA, eds. *Current Practice of Clinical Electroencephalography.* 3rd ed. Lippincott Williams & Wilkins, Philadelphia, 2003:288–302.

Epileptiform Abnormalities

WILLIAM O. TATUM, IV

SELIM R. BENBADIS

Interictal epileptiform discharges (IED) represent a distinctive group of waveforms that are characteristically seen in persons with epilepsy. Variations of normal background rhythms, a variety of artifacts, and variants of uncertain significance may mimic abnormal IEDs and lead to overinterpretation of the EEG (Chapter 1). IEDs have reliably been associated with epilepsy at rates sufficient enough to be clinically useful. Although prominent intrapatient and interpatient variability in morphology may occur, those with the most pronounced spikes on EEG are not necessarily associated with a greater severity of epilepsy. Scalp detection of IEDs is based upon dipole localization and the surrounding field, although it may be different than the site of seizure genesis. In most cases, an IED will reflect radial oriented dipoles detected on the scalp, however in other situations, tangential dipoles from individual epilepsy syndromes (benign childhood epilepsy with centrotemporal spikes [BCECTS]) or developmentally or surgically altered cortex may create unusual dipoles that produce challenging patterns to the EEG reader. Rarely, normal individuals may possess IEDs on EEG without the phenotypic expression of seizures. The photoparoxysmal response, generalized spike-and-wave, or centrotemporal IEDs are most frequently encountered, and may represent idiopathic, genetically acquired traits that are represented on EEG without the expression of seizures. Focal IEDs may have a variable association with the clinical epilepsy depending upon location. For example, central, parietal, and occipital spikes, in general, are more benign regions than frontal and temporal locations and have a relatively reduced potential for epileptogenicity in the absence of a structural lesion.

The interictal EEG has a pivotal role in providing ancillary support for a clinical diagnosis of epilepsy (seizure disorder). In EEG, IEDs may help classify the epilepsy or epilepsy syndrome by identifying IEDs in conjunction with the clinical semiology. Classification of the epilepsies are based upon distinguishing seizures that are localization-related from those that are generalized by the type and distribution of IEDs noted on the EEG. Focal IEDs may be either focal, regional, lateralized, or secondarily generalized discharges in their field of involvement. They may help provide information useful in localizing the epileptogenic zone for the purposes of surgical treatment. Frontal, anterior temporal, and midline IEDs have the highest correlation with seizures. Furthermore, there is treatment information that can be clinically relevant following therapy (i.e., as in the case of absence seizures), in addition to prognosticating when a trial of antiepileptic drug taper is planned by providing information about persistent IEDs on EEG. In the absence of IEDs, epilepsy is not excluded because of the deep cortex, fissures, gryi, and sulcal neuroanatomy that may not readily be represented at the scalp during routine recording. The EEG, while ideally suited for evaluating patients with epilepsy, is also not specific for etiology when demonstrating IEDs. The scalp EEG may demonstrate both interictal and ictal (Chapter 4) discharges in the same or different regions of the brain.

FOCAL EPILEPTIFORM DISCHARGES

Abnormal focal interictal epileptiform discharges on EEG represent a heightened predisposition for the expression of partial-onset seizures. The location of focal interictal epileptiform discharges vary with respect to the potential to generate clinical seizures and also the behavioral manifestations that are likely to occur.

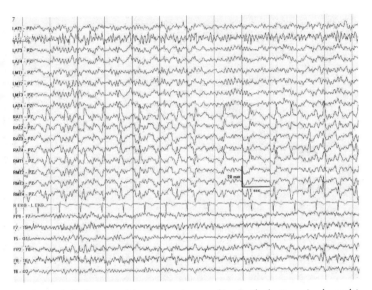

FIGURE 3.1. Intracranial versus scalp recording (in the bottom six channels) during a presurgical evaluation of intractable epilepsy. Sensitivities in the top channels are 75 μv versus 7 μv/mm at the scalp. Note the absence of IEDs in the scalp EEG compared to the intracranial EEG where they occur at 1/sec.

It is often said that a normal interictal EEG does not exclude a clinical diagnosis of epilepsy. The cortex sampled by surface-based *scalp EEG* is an incomplete representation of the entire brain. Many deep-seated cortical gyri are unable to be "seen" unless intracranial electrodes are placed directly over the underlying cortex. Because scalp potentials are volume-conducted potentials through cerebrospinal fluid and meninges, skull, and subcutaneous tissue of the scalp, "buried" or low-amplitude potentials may be underrepresented at the level of scalp recording. Therefore, difficulty with source detection at the level of the scalp may arise because of deep-seated foci (i.e., mesial frontal), small restricted foci, rapid cortical spread, or obscuration by movement or myogenic artifact.

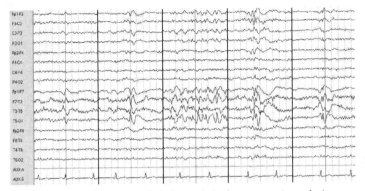

FIGURE 3.2. Different morphologies include sharp waves (seen during seconds 1 and 2), spikes and sharp waves (in second 3), polyspike-and-slow waves (in second 4), and spike-and-wave discharges (in the last second of the figure) recorded during an ambulatory EEG in a patient with epilepsy.

Epileptiform discharges appear in different morphologies. Commonly identified IEDs are spikes and sharp waves with or without aftergoing slow waves. *Polyspikes* (or multispikes) are also IEDs. Note a single sharp wave in the first second and a spike-and-slow wave complex in the last second. Both *spikes* and *sharp waves* are referred to as interictal epileptiform discharges (transients). Sharp waves are more "blunted" than spikes and are IEDs with a duration of 70 to 200 msec. Combinations of IEDs often occur in the same patient at different times (see Figure 3.2 above). Both spikes and sharp waves are generated at the top of the cortical gyrus and have a polarity that is most often negative at the surface of the scalp recording.

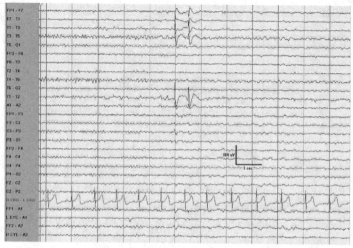

FIGURE 3.3. EEG demonstrating a couplet of left anterior temporal spike-and-slow waves.

Focal interictal epileptiform discharges (IEDs) suggest a partial mechanism exists in a patient with a clinical diagnosis of epilepsy or seizures. The polarity of an abnormal epileptiform discharge designated as a spike, is very frequently negative at the surface of the scalp EEG. The duration is 20 to 70 msec. Those discharges of <20 msec are suspect for noncerebral potentials. There may or may not be an aftergoing slow wave discharge. The location usually determines the potential for epileptogenicity with temporal locations usually carrying the highest association with clinical seizure expression. Furthermore, the seizure semiology can be inferred with anterior temporal IEDs carrying a greater risk for the expression of complex partial seizures of temporal lobe origin.

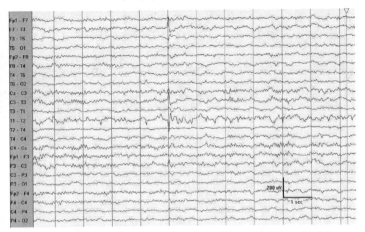

FIGURE 3.4. Left temporal sharp waves in a 43-year-old man after left temporal lobectomy evaluated for reoperation. Note the positive phase reversal at T3.

Positive spikes are rarely encountered in the EEG. Interictal epileptiform discharges (spikes and sharp waves) are almost always surface negative, generating the typical negative phase reversal. The situation encountered most commonly in clinical practice in which they may have a positive polarity is in patients who have had surgery and altered cortical anatomy. In neonatal EEG, positive IEDs reflect periventricular injury and are not uncommon, although with development, unless congenital brain malformations are evident, positive sharp waves are rarely encountered.

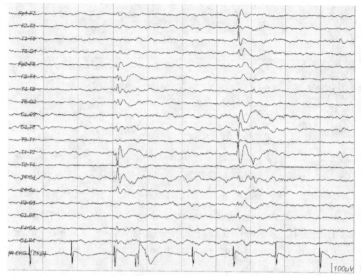

FIGURE 3.5. Bilateral anterior temporal sharp-and-slow wave in drowsiness.

The location varies with the site of epileptogenicity but is commonly seen in the temporal regions. Anterior temporal spikes or sharp waves often have a clinical association with complex partial seizures of temporal lobe origin more than 90% of the time. These discharges have maximal electronegativity at the F7/F8 derivations using the 10–20 system of electrode placement. However, the amplitude of these IEDs is usually greatest in the "true temporal" (at T1 and T2), ear, or sphenoidal electrodes when these electrodes are utilized. In one-third of patients, the discharges are seen bilaterally, are activated by sleep, and localize best in wakefulness or rapid eye movement (REM) sleep when present.

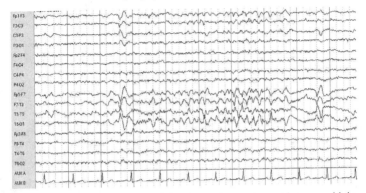

FIGURE 3.6. Left mid-temporal sharp wave in a patient with temporal lobe epilepsy. Note the focal theta and delta slowing regionally in the same region.

Mid-temporal IEDs also occur in patients with temporal lobe epilepsy (TLE). In general, mid-temporal IEDs are often more regional in distribution with neocortical TLE. Focal slowing and the presence of bilateral discharges appear more likely to be equally represented.

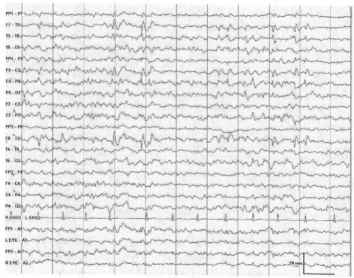

FIGURE 3.7. Left centroemporal spikes in a patient with BCECTS. Notice the central field of spread of the spikes and low-amplitude right frontal positivity.

Benign childhood epilepsy with centrotemporal spikes (BCECTS; also called rolandic epilepsy) is a common childhood idiopathic localization-related epilepsy syndrome. In this case, a contralateral positive phase reversal may appear in the contralateral frontal region characterizing the tangential dipole of BCECTS. The sharp waves have a characteristic diphasic morphology with a negative peak followed by a positive rounded component that is markedly activated during non-REM sleep.

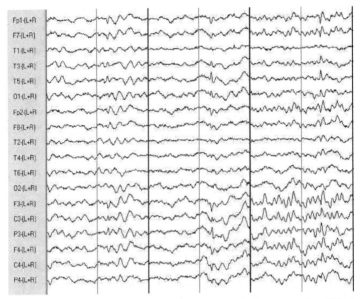

FIGURE 3.8. The same spikes depicted in Figure 3.7 demonstrated on linked ears reference montage. Note the frontal positivity denoting the tangential dipole of BCECTs.

The characteristic tangential or horizontal dipole that is formed in BCECTs demonstrates both a negativity and positivity during the discharge. This has been used to separate the more "benign" nature of BCECTs from a more pathological rolandic sharp wave. This dipole characteristically reveals a maximum negativity in the centrotemporal region and a contralateral maximum positivity in the frontal (or vertex) region that is best demonstrated on referential montages.

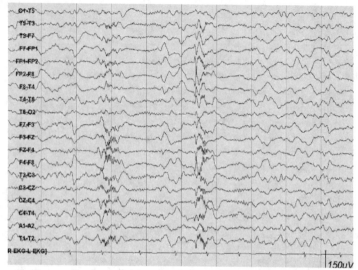

FIGURE 3.9. A right frontal spike and polyspike discharge in frontal lobe epilepsy.

Frontal spikes are often found in patients with frontal lobe epilepsy (FLE), although they may be absent in up to one-third of patients. They may also appear as fragmented generalized spike-and-wave discharges in idiopathic generalized epilepsy (IGE) during drowsiness. The IEDs of FLE are often spikes with high-amplitude broad discharges that may be reflected in the contralateral frontal region. Secondary bilateral synchrony (SBS) or diffuse discharges arising from a focal point in the frontal lobe may occur in up to two-thirds of individuals with FLE. Transverse montages are best to distinguish a lateralized generator from two discrete bisynchronous generators.

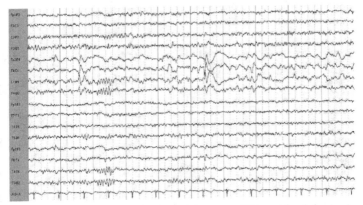

FIGURE 3.10. Right central spike-and-slow wave IEDs and focal slowing in a patient with a right frontal tumor and partial seizures.

Central IEDs can occur with the symptomatic localization-related epilepsy (LREs) at any age. Overall, central IEDs are less frequently associated with epilepsy than those arising from temporal or frontal lobe origin. Some conditions may give rise to central spikes without epilepsy and include cerebral palsy, migraine, and inherited trait without seizures (i.e., siblings of those with BCECTS), and normal variants (i.e., fragmented mu rhythm). Unlike normal rhythms (i.e., mu rhythms), central IEDs often have a quicker "rise" on the upstroke of the discharge, may be associated with an aftergoing slow wave, occur in a state independent fashion (not just drowsiness and light sleep), and/or be associated with focal slowing in the same region.

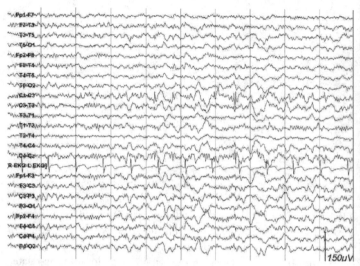

FIGURE 3.11. Midline spikes and polyspikes in a patient with frontal lobe epilepsy.

Midline spikes may occur at Cz, Fz, and Pz and are seen more frequently in children but may also occur in adults. Isolated midline spikes, polyspikes, or pathological sharp waves are most often noted at the central vertex, and have a high association with epilepsy. No distinct clinical syndrome exists for patients with midline spikes. Tonic seizures are the most frequent seizure type. In patients with Pz spikes or parietal lobe epilepsy, scalp EEG is often of limited yield or demonstrates falsely localizing abnormalities including IEDs in the temporal or frontal regions.

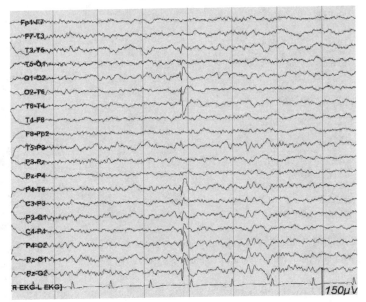

FIGURE 3.12. A single right occipital spike-and-slow wave discharge shown in both a bipolar and reference montage (last two channels).

Occipital IEDs are most frequently reported in the benign childhood epilepsies with occipital paroxysms and the later-onset Panayiotopoulos syndrome. Occipital spikes may appear in nonepileptic patients who express the IEDs as a genetic trait, or those who are congenitally blind ("needle spikes" of the blind). Occipital IEDs have been noted in children with visual dysfunction and benign occipital epilepsies and in adults with structural lesions and symptomatic occipital lobe epilepsy with or without a visual aura.

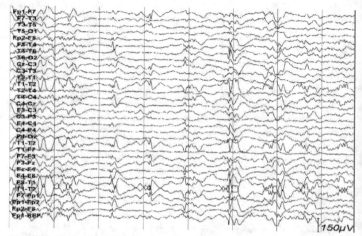

FIGURE 3.13. Multifocal independent spike discharges seen in a patient with encephalopathic generalized epilepsy.

Multifocal spikes may be seen in individuals with discrete structural lesions, although usually they are associated with diffuse structural injury involving the gray matter of the hemispheres. Mental retardation and cerebral palsy are common underlying substrates for patients with multifocal independent spike discharges. There may be a primary site of focal dysfunction or be associated with concomitant generalized epileptiform discharges such as with the Lennox-Gastaut syndrome.

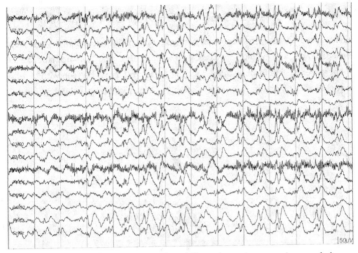

FIGURE 3.14. A burst of secondary bilateral synchronous burst of sharp-and-slow waves. Note the left frontotemporal spikes prior to the burst.

S*econdary bilateral synchrony* (SBS) is a term used for a generalized discharge with a focal onset. These diffuse bursts are best distinguished when a "lead in" of 400 msec or more is noted in a patient with independent focal IEDs. Patients with medial frontal seizures such as those with supplementary motor area, medial frontal convexity, or cingulate gyrus area involvement are most likely to manifest SBS given their proximity to the corpus callosum. IEDs or slowing may be best seen independently over the frontal and frontal-polar regions when orbital frontal seizures occur. Midline EEG electrodes with vertex representation are important to detect discharges in this region.

GENERALIZED EPILEPTIFORM DISCHARGES

Generalized epileptiform discharges are typically seen in patients with generalized epilepsy and are helpful to classify the idiopathic and symptomatic forms. Generalized epileptiform discharges vary in duration and may be seen with or without clinical signs or even appear less often as an inherited trait without seizures.

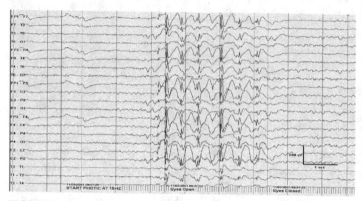

FIGURE 3.15. Self-limited photoparoxysmal response in a patient without seizures evaluated for headaches.

A photoparoxysmal (PPR) or photoconvulsive response consists of a burst of generalized spikes and/or polyspike-and-slow wave complexes provoked by photic stimulation. The most frequent provocative frequencies appear around 15 Hz (see Figure 3.15 above). Eye closure may evoke the PPR and is performed during intermittent photic stimulation (IPS). It has a clinical correlation with idiopathic generalized epilepsy (IGE), although it may also appear as an inherited trait without seizures. A non–self-limited PPR beyond the duration of the stimulus has been more frequently associated with epilepsy according to some investigators.

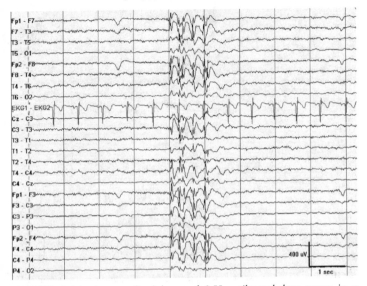

FIGURE 3.16. A generalized burst of 3-Hz spike-and-slow waves in a patient with IGE and absence seizures.

The prototypic abnormality on EEG seen with generalized seizures is the 3-Hz spike-and-slow-wave complex. It appears as a bilateral, synchronous, symmetrical, surface-negative spike maximal in the frontal-central regions, followed by a surface-negative slow wave in a longitudinal bipolar montage. Minor lateralized asymmetry may be observed. Response times may be impaired regardless of burst duration, although longer bursts imply longer periods of impaired responsiveness. Alerting responses inhibit generalized spike-and-wave (GSW), while sleep, hyperventilation, and intermittent photic stimulation often increase it in IGE. In sleep, the bursts of GSW may "fragment," and appear irregular and lateralized, having a slower repetitition rate and a greater predisposition to polyspike formation.

89

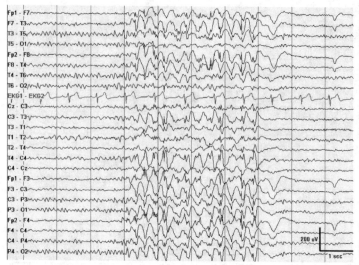

FIGURE 3.17. A burst of generalized 3.5-Hz spike-and-slow waves in JME.

Spike-and-slow-wave complexes that have a repetition rate of >3 Hz are referred to as *fast GSW*. JME is the most common idiopathic generalized epilepsy (IGE) syndrome associated with myoclonus and often demonstrates fast spike-and-slow wave complexes with frequencies of 3.5 to 5.0 Hz on the interictal EEG that may slow to 2.25 to 2.5 Hz during longer bursts. However, "typical" 3-Hz GSW may be seen in 25% of individuals with juvenile myoclonic epilepsy (JME). Focal features may also occur during seizures, as well as on EEG, although they probably represent fragmentation of the generalized discharge in the majority of cases.

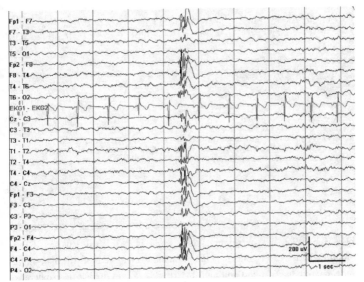

FIGURE 3.18. Generalized polyspike-and-slow wave in a patient with JME.

The most characteristic feature on EEG in patients with JME is generalized, bisynchronous, frontocentral predominant "fast" polyspike-and-slow wave (PSW) complexes, although this may also be seen in other IGEs as well. The discharges are maximal in the frontal regions with two or more high-voltage surface-negative spikes best described as polyspikes (or multispikes). The incidence of the PSW bursts increases on awakening and frequently translates to early morning myoclonus or generalized tonic-clonic (GTC) seizures. Sleep deprivation is a potent activator of the generalized IEDs seen with JME. Photosensitivity may occur in up to 40% of patients with JME and is more prominent in females.

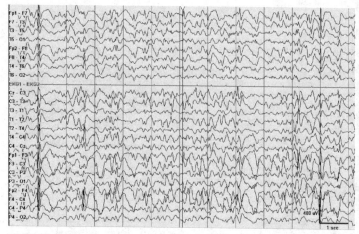

FIGURE 3.19. Hypsarrhythmia in a child with infantile spasms that is "modified" due to a right congenital brain malformation. Note the high-amplitude, chaotic background and multifocal spikes within the left hemisphere.

Hypsarrhythmia is a distinctive pattern that is seen in children and often associated with infantile spasms as a manifestation of West syndrome. A high-voltage background composed of disorganized slow theta and delta frequencies is seen in addition to nearly continuous multi-focal interictal epileptiform discharges. Modified patterns are noted with variations in amplitude and hemispheric predominance and may occur with attenuations that may correlate with infantile spasms. Many patients with hypsarrhythmia evolve into the pattern of diffuse slowing, multifocal IEDs, and slow-spike-and-waves characteristic of the Lennox-Gastaut syndrome.

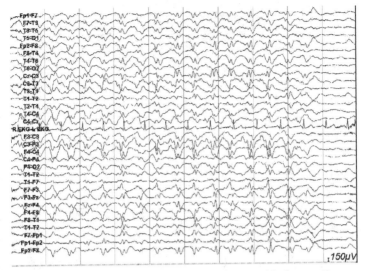

FIGURE 3.20. Slow-spike-and-wave in a patient with Lennox-Gastaut syndrome.

Slow-spike(or sharp)-and-wave discharges (SSW) are <3 Hz and are present in patients with the Lennox-Gastaut syndrome (LGS). This most often consists of a biphasic or triphasic surface- negative sharp wave followed by a slow wave in a bilateral, synchronous, symmetrical, frontocentral complex. They often appear as repetitive bursts or runs of frequencies ranging from 1.5 to 2.5 Hz and often asymmetrical or shifting and prolonged in sleep. These IEDs are not activated with either hyperventilation (HV) or IPS. A less discrete onset and offset with a longer duration is seen with the SSW discharges as opposed to that seen with "typical" 3-Hz GSW discharges. In addition to the characteristic SSW, patients with LGS may manifest focal or multifocal epileptiform discharges. Most SSW bursts are interictal, although atypical absence seizures are the most ictal correlate seen.

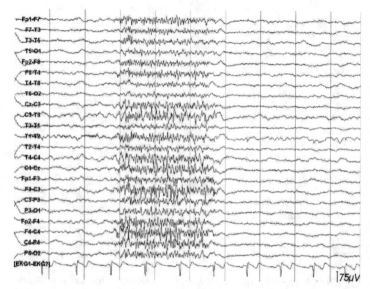

FIGURE 3.21. An asymptomatic burst of GPFA in a patient with the Lennox-Gastaut syndrome and tonic seizures.

Generalized paroxysmal fast activity (GPFA) is another feature on EEG that occurs with the slow spike-and-waves of LGS. It is primarily seen during sleep and consists of diffuse, bilateral bursts of 15 to 20 Hz frontally predominant bursts of fast frequencies. Variable frequencies, voltages, and durations may occur, although they usually last several seconds. This feature frequently has no overtly detectable clinical manifestations, although it may correlate with tonic seizures when occurring while awake or with durations of >6 sec.

ADDITIONAL RESOURCES

Abraham K, Ajmone-Marsan C. Patterns of cortical discharges and their relation to routine scalp electroencephalography. *Electroencephalogr Clin Neurophysiol Suppl* 1958;10:447–461.

Ebersole JS. Defining epileptogenic foci: past, present, and future. *J Clin Neurophysiol* 1997;14:470–483.

Gregory RP, Oates T, Merry RT. Electroencephalogram epileptiform abnormalities in candidates for aircrew training. *Electroencephalogr Clin Neurophysiol* 1993;86:75–77.

Maulsby RL. Some guidelines for the assessment of spikes and sharp waves in EEG tracings. *Am J EEG Technol* 1971;11:3–16.

Pedley TA, Mendiratta A, Walczak TS. Seizures and epilepsy. In: Ebersole JS, Pedley TA, eds. *Current Practice of Clinical Electroencephalography*. 3rd ed. Lippincott Williams & Wilkins, Philadelphia, 2003:506–587.

Pillai J, Sperling MR. Interictal EEG and the diagnosis of epilepsy. Epilepsia 2006;47(Suppl. 1):14–22.

Shewmon DA, Erwin RJ. The effect of focal interictal spikes on perception of reaction time. I. General considerations. *Electroencephalogr Clin Neurophysiol* 1988;69:319–377.

Tao JX, Ray A, Hawes-Ebersole S, Ebersole JS. Incracranial EEG substrates of scalp EEG interictal spikes. *Epilepsia* 2005;46(5):669–676.

Seizures

PETER W. KAPLAN

WILLIAM O. TATUM, IV

The EEG is able to provide a definitive diagnosis of epilepsy when seizures are recorded. Additionally, classification of the seizure type for the purposes of identifying the type of epilepsy to direct treatment can be deduced. These ictal patterns may serve as the basis for localization of recurrent seizures in epilepsy that are useful not only in the diagnosis but also in the treatment selection and prognosis. The EEG provides only supportive evidence for a clinical diagnosis of epilepsy when interictal epileptiform discharges are present because unless a seizure is recorded IEDs may appear without associated seizures. For focal seizures, there are a wide variety of EEG expression affecting frequency, amplitude, distribution, rhythmicity, and evolution. Ictal discharges are most frequently composed of repetitive rhythmic frequencies as opposed to simple repetition of interictal epileptiform discharges. Generalized onset seizures are more stereotyped. Furthermore, the EEG may indicate electrographic evidence of seizures even in the absence of a clinical correlate in situations of states of altered awareness when continuous or repetitive seizures occur that are not convulsive and overtly visible to others. Monitoring status epilepticus during treatment as well as monitoring EEG in the intensive care unit, critical care unit, or emergency department may provide clinical input relative to the presence, quantity, and response to treatment when seizures or status epilepticus is considered. There is an interictal-ictal transition that is best defined as a continuum. This chapter will provide the seizure types and their associated EEG findings.

GENERALIZED SEIZURES

Generalized seizures have a homogeneous clinical behavior compared to focal seizures. In idiopathic generalized epilepsy, several seizure types may overlap and appear as epilepsy syndromes. Generalized seizures associated with symptomatic generalized epilepsy are more heterogeneous but are characteristic of patients with diffuse structural injury.

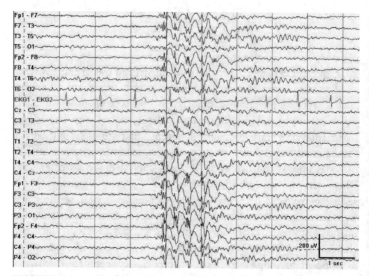

FIGURE 4.1. A brief 1-sec burst of 3-Hz generalized polyspike-spike-and-wave that is associated with a "postictal" arousal.

Most generalized spike-and-wave discharges that are shorter than 3 sec in duration *do not* typically demonstrate clinically noticeable signs. However, even a single spike-and-wave discharge may be associated with a subtle behavioral alteration of responsiveness that is not clinically discernible with gross testing modalities. Notice the change in alerting seen after the 1-sec burst of generalized spike and polyspike-and-waves in the above figure.

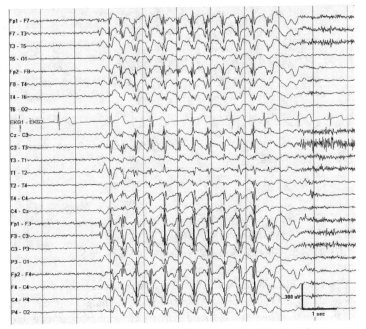

FIGURE 4.2. Absence seizure. Note the asymmetrical left frontal onset.

The 3-Hz spike-and-wave pattern is suggestive of idiopathic generalized epilepsy. When bursts of 3-Hz spike-and-waves are generalized, regular, symmetrical, synchronous, and maximal in the anterior head regions and are longer than 3 sec, the EEG strongly suggests the diagnosis of absence seizure (petit mal). During sleep, absence seizures may become more irregular and longer in duration. In addition, like the seizure semiology, the EEG may show assymetries or lateralizing features during absence seizures (see above). With aging, absence seizures may become more irregular and slower in frequency.

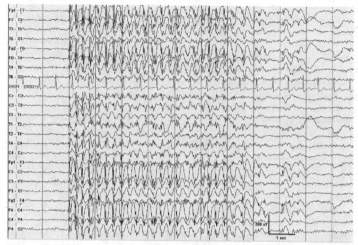

FIGURE 4.3. Absence (petit mal) seizure in an 8-year-old boy.

During an absence seizure, the EEG demonstrates generalized, regular, synchronous 3-Hz spike-and-wave discharges in the setting of waking or drowsy background activity. These discharges may start at a rate of >3 Hz, but eventually slow down to a discharge frequency slightly above 2 Hz. Maximum amplitude is in the fronto-central region, often with phase reversals bilaterally at F3 and F4. In some patients, the spike component may be subtle or absent, and replaced by rhythmic slow activity. When prolonged bursts of generalized spike-and-waves (GSW) last >3 sec, impaired responsiveness is likely to become clinically evident. Shifting asymmetries are not unusual and do not constitute a focal onset.

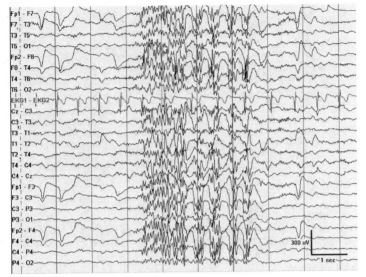

FIGURE 4.4. Atypical absence seizure in a patient with encephalopathic generalized epilepsy. Notice the polyspikes that evolve to a slow spike-and-wave pattern.

Atypical absence seizures are clinically similar to typical absence seizures seen in Figures 4.2 and 4.3; however, they may have more incomplete loss of awareness or responsiveness. On the EEG, the bursts often have a more gradual onset and offset. Slow spike-and-wave bursts accompany atypical absence seizures and have a <2.5-Hz frequency in the awake state and may have sharp waves or polyspikes prior to the aftergoing slow wave (see above). There are frequent asymmetries and are often associated interictal epileptiform discharges (IEDs) that may be multifocal.

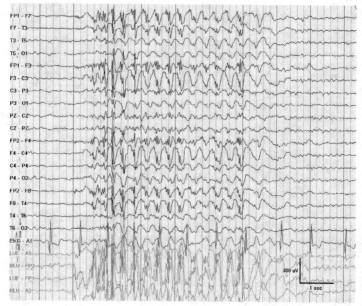

FIGURE 4.5. Myoclonic seizure associated with a burst of generalized poly-spike-and-waves in a patient with juvenile myoclonic epilepsy (JME).

Myoclonic seizures are associated with a single complex or burst of generalized spike or polyspike-and-waves. The polyspike formation is evident in the example above and is associated with myoclonus at the onset of this seizure. Isolated polyspike-and-wave discharges may be associated with myoclonus that is obscured by an overriding artifact. Extracerebral electrodes may become helpful to distinguish myogenic spikes from that of polyspike IEDs.

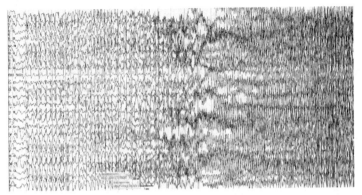

FIGURE 4.6. Myoclonus followed by generalized tonic-clonic seizure in a patient with JME.

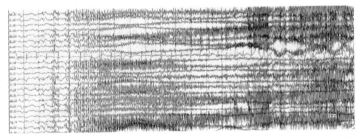

FIGURE 4.7. This seizure represented a tonic-clonic seizure in a patient with IGE and recurrent generalized seizures on awakening.

Generalized tonic-clonic (GTC), or "grand mal" seizures, are generalized seizures with a tonic and clonic component. The EEG demonstrates a "recruiting rhythm" that is composed of repetitive alpha frequencies in the maximal anterior head regions. Initial myogenic artifact obscures the record prior to the decrescendo phasic movement artifact of the clonic phase that gradually stops prior to generalized post-ictal suppression on the EEG. The GTC seizure may be seen in idiopathic generalized epilepsy (IGE) without a focal onset, or become secondarily generalized from a focal origin. Lateralized or focal features suggest the latter situation.

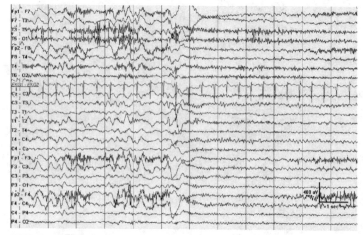

FIGURE 4.8. Infantile spasm noted in second 7 above with an electrodecremental response obtained in a 3-year-old child with tuberous sclerosis. Note the high amplitude.

Infantile spasms are brief tonic spasms that involve head flexion and arm abduction and extension for seconds, usually occurring in clusters between 1 and 3 years of age. There are several forms that may occur depending upon the degree of somatic involvement, and are typically associated with mental impairment. The spasms begin with an abrupt generalized electrodecremental response on EEG with generalized attenuation of the background frequencies which may have faster frequencies superimposed lasting from <1 sec to several seconds.

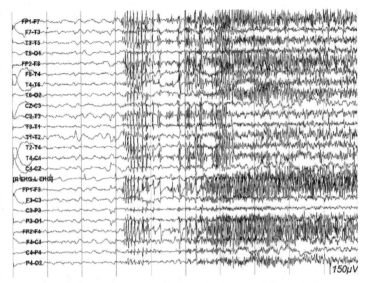

FIGURE 4.9. Tonic seizure in a patient with Lennox-Gastaut syndrome.

Tonic seizures are associated with symptomatic generalized epilepsy and are the most common seizure type associated with the Lennox-Gastaut syndrome. Tonic seizures typically have an abrupt onset of a generalized 10-Hz rhythm on EEG. Generalized paroxysmal fast activity is often seen as the associated features on EEG, although it may have no apparent clinical features associated with brief bursts that occur during sleep. Low-voltage fast frequencies associated with a generalized attenuation of the background may also be evident during a tonic seizure.

FOCAL SEIZURES

Focal seizures have a wide variety of EEG abnormalities that may occur depending upon the location of the epileptogenic zone generating the ictal discharge. Some focal seizures have no detectable representation at the surface of the scalp recorded EEG. Furthermore, some focal seizures have an ictal pattern that is diffuse and appear falsely "generalized" in distribution or even appear with subtle or without detectable clinical features.

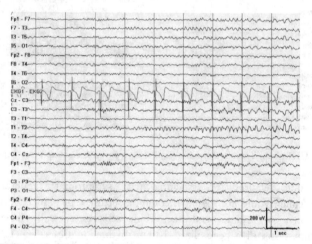

FIGURE 4.10. The above EEG shows a simple partial seizure that occurred out of stage 2 sleep.

Simple partial seizures are partial seizures that do not involve impairment of consciousness and when associated with clinical features reflect the aura. Most patients with mesial temporal lobe epilepsy report an aura. However, while auras are nonspecific, experiential, or viscerosensory symptoms including rising epigastric sensations, "butterflies," nausea, fear, and deja vu are common. Despite the presence of clinical symptoms, auras may be detected by scalp EEG only approximately 40% of the time on routine recording.

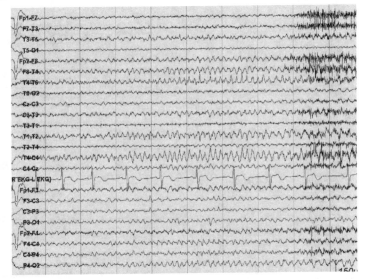

FIGURE 4.11. Right temporal 6- to 7-Hz rhythmic ictal theta discharge at seizure onset in a patient with temporal lobe epilepsy.

Mesial temporal lobe seizures are the most common adult seizure type, presenting as a complex partial seizure that involve impairment of consciousness. Interictal EEG manifestations include anterior temporal spikes at 0.5 to 1.5 Hz or rhythmic 2 to 4 Hz facilitated by drowsiness and light non-REM sleep. A frequent ictal pattern of mesial temporal origin is the sudden appearance of localized or regional background attenuation, build-up of 4- to 7-Hz rhythmic activity, increasing in amplitude as it slows to 1 to 2 Hz. This may be followed by suppression or slow activity.

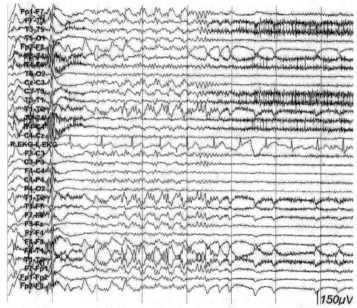

FIGURE 4.12. Left temporal neocortical seizure onset with rhythmic 3-Hz delta maximal in the mid-temporal derivation prior to rapid generalization.

Lateral or neocortical temporal seizures differ from those that begin in the mesial portion of the temporal lobe. Although it may be difficult to clinically distinguish neocortical temporal lobe seizures from mesial temporal lobe seizures, they may have a widespread hemispheric onset, begin in the mid-temporal derivations at <5 Hz, have rapid propagation to extratemporal structures, and have a greater likelihood to secondarily generalize as seen above. It is also not uncommon to have a bilateral ictal onset noted on EEG with neo-cortical temporal lobe seizure onset.

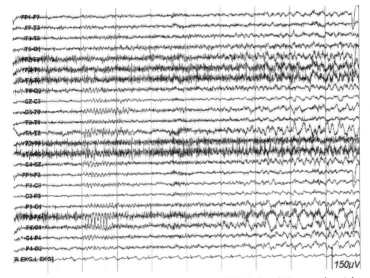

FIGURE 4.13. Temporal lobe seizure onset falsely localizing to the right frontal region on scalp EEG. Note the initial alpha frequencies that persist in the theta range.

Some patients with temporal lobe epilepsy (TLE) may have projected rhythms to the anterior head regions. In the above example, a right anterior temporal lobe lesion was seen and created the appearance of a right frontal discharge initially present as a burst of repetitive spikes that evolved to an irregular right fronto-temporal theta rhythm. The patient has been seizure free after right temporal lobectomy for 2 years.

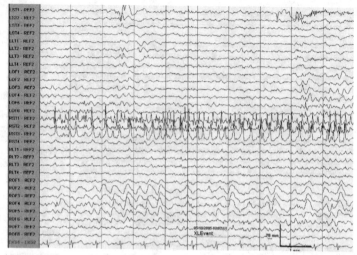

FIGURE 4.14. Right "focal" temporal seizure confined to the right subtemporal (RST) 1 to 3 electrodes on intracranial recording. L(R)ST = left (right) subtemporal; L(R)LT = left (right) lateral temporal; L(R)OF = left (right) orbitofrontal.

Partial seizures may originate from one to two electrodes at seizure onset. Those seizures with a "focal" origin on the intracranial EEG imply a restricted generator adjacent to the recording electrode. In Figure 4.14, RST1 demonstrated an abrupt onset of rhythmic ictal frequencies >13 Hz prior to RST1-3 repetitive spiking that remained a well-localized unilateral discharge for 20 sec prior to contralateral involvement of the left hemisphere. The "focal" onset, location, and prolonged unilateral involvement prior to propagation are favorable features for localizing seizures onset. Following right temporal lobectomy, the patient has remained seizure free.

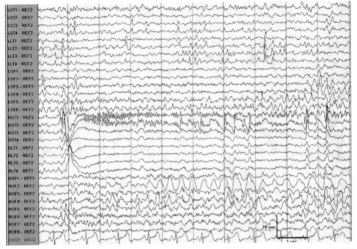

FIGURE 4.15. Right "regional" temporal onset noted in the RST and RLT subdural strip electrodes. L(R)ST = left (right) subtemporal; L(R)LT = left (right) lateral temporal; L(R)OF = left (right) orbitofrontal.

Regional onsets in patients with temporal lobe epilepsy identified by intracranial electrodes demonstrate more widespread areas of ictal onset. Lateralization and regionalization of the ictal activity are then complementary to the remaining parameters of the presurgical evaluation to demonstrate concordance for the purposes of epilepsy surgery. In the above EEG, note the large sharply contoured slow wave and regional attenuation in the RST and RLT strips and rhythmic ictal fast activity in RST 1 and 2 at seizure onset.

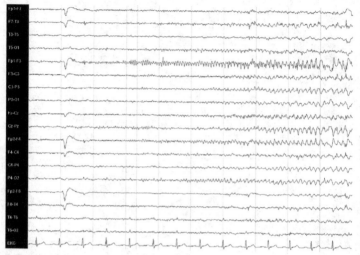

FIGURE 4.16. Discrete focal seizure onset in a patient with a right frontal lesion. (Courtesy of Imran Ali, MD.)

Frequently because much of the frontal lobe is underrepresented by scalp electrodes, ictal recordings in frontal lobe epilepsy are associated with nonlocalized and often nonlateralized ictal EEG on scalp recording. Anterior and dorsolateral onset may be associated with focal IEDs and even focal electrographic seizures, although this is typically observed when scalp ictal EEG changes are evident. Note the infrequently seen focal ictal onset in the patient above with lesional frontal lobe epilepsy evident at FP1.

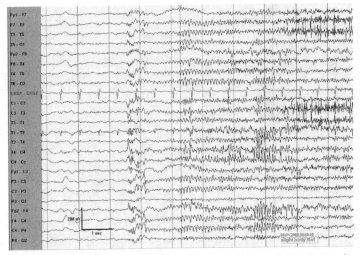

FIGURE 4.17. Nonlocalized ictal EEG in frontal lobe epilepsy. Notice the brief right frontal-central repetitive spikes in seconds 7 to 8.

Frontal lobe epilepsy often has very brief, bizarre, bimanual-bipedal automatisms with nocturnal predominance and be prone to acute repetitive seizures and status epilepticus. It is the second more common location in large epilepsy surgery series. Ictal scalp EEG is often of limited utility. In orbitofrontal and mesial frontal onset, seizures may have no representation at all or be obscured by an over-riding muscle artifact to make scalp EEG "invisible" during the seizure. Interictal epileptiform discharges are notably absent in 30% of patients with frontal lobe epilepsy. Orbitofrontal and mesial frontal may not manifest interictal or even ictal discharges at all. Midline electrodes are crucial in cases of mesial frontal origin.

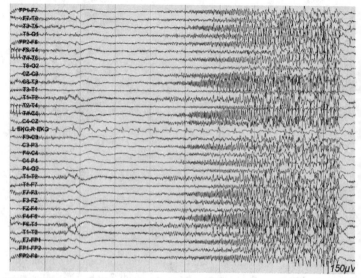

FIGURE 4.18. Diffuse electrodecremental response in a patient with a supplementary motor seizure.

Supplementary motor seizures are seizures that begin in the mesial frontal lobe and therefore often may have brief and bizarre semiologies that mimic psychogenic nonepileptic seizures (pseudo-pseudoseizures). The clinical semiology may also manifest a "fencer's" posture that provides more localizing value than surface ictal EEG (see above) with the side of tonic extension reflecting the side opposite seizure onset.

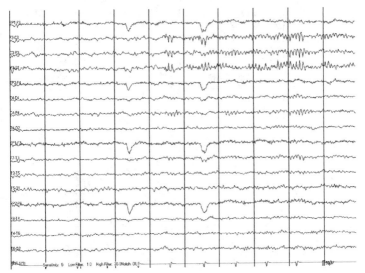

FIGURE 4.19. The tracing shows high-frequency, mu-like arcuate waveforms focally over the left parietal C3-P3 derivations at 10 Hz in the region of a brain tumor.

Parietal lobe seizures are often clinically silent. Somatosensory involvement may yield a perception of tingling, formication, pain, heat, movement, or dysmorphopsia, typically of the distal limb or face. As in frontal lobe epilepsy, only a small number of those with parietal ictal onset are focal. Spread may occur to the supplementary motor area or temporal area and result in electrographic lateralization or even localization late in the seizure onset. The patient above noted paroxysmal right arm and leg tingling during the recording.

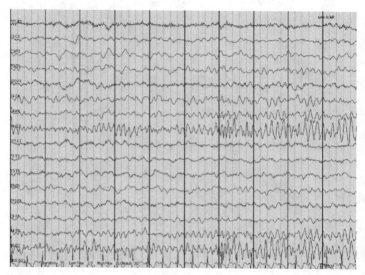

FIGURE 4.20. Right occipital lobe seizure with a build-up of right occipital 6- to 7-Hz rhythmic ictal theta associated with the patient's complaint of left visual field loss.

Occipital lobe seizures commonly manifest phosphenes, unformed visual hallucinations, and less frequently blindness and hemianopsia. There may be illusions that objects appear larger (macropsia), smaller (micropsia), distorted (metamorphopsia), or persistent after the visual stimulus (pallinopsia). High-frequency discharges at the temporoparieto-occipital junction can induce contraversive nystagmus and eye and head deviation. The EEG may show build-up of rapid alpha-beta activity focally over the temporoparieto-occipital junction or more posteriorly (see above), often with spread anteriorly to temporal structures as the seizure progresses from simple partial to complex partial semiology.

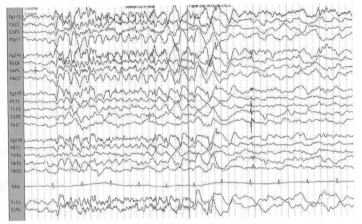

FIGURE 4.21. Subclinical seizure in a patient with encephalopathic generalized epilepsy. There were no clinical signs noted during multiple brief seizures.

Subclinical seizures are an artifact of testing with the degree of "subclinical" occurrence reflecting the sophistication of behavioral testing. Seizures may occur without awareness or be very subtle such that clinical signs are not noted. These are especially common in patients with complex partial seizures. When testing is performed, some seizures exhibit no evidence of interruption in behavior. Such is the case with brief absence seizures. In the patient above with encephalopathic generalized epilepsy, the seizures were unassociated with any clinical signs despite behavioral testing (counting).

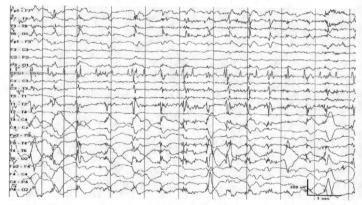

FIGURE 4.22. Multiple electrode artifacts simulating IEDs in a patient with psychogenic non-epileptic seizures (PNES).

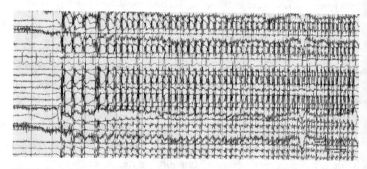

FIGURE 4.23. "Ictal" EEG in a PNES. Note the evolution of the rhythmic myogenic artifact that occurred with repetitive jaw movement mimicking an epileptic seizure.

As expected, the EEG during a nonepileptic seizure is normal. The importance of defining seizures as epileptic or nonepileptic is reflected in the number of patients with PNES. While the precise incidence is undefined, they account for 20% to 25% of admissions to hospital- based epilepsy monitoring units and are about as prevalent as multiple sclerosis.

Overinterpretation of EEG patterns that are normal is a common substrate for misdiagnosis. An artifact may also be the culprit leading to a false diagnosis of epilepsy, as in the example above (compare the similarity in "pseudoevolution" to Figure 4.7).

ADDITIONAL RESOURCES

Benbadis SR. The EEG of nonepileptic seizures. *J Clin Neurophsyiol* 2006;23: 340–352.

Blume WT, Holloway GM, Wiebe S. Temporal epileptogenesis: localizing value of scalp and subdural interictal and ictal EEG data. *Epilepsia* 2000;42:508–514.

Farrell K, Tatum WO. Enecphalopathic generalized epilepsy and Lennox-Gastaut syndrome. In: Wyllie E, ed. *The Treatment of Epilepsy; Practice and Principals.* 4th ed. Baltimore, Lippincott Williams & Williams, 2006:429–440.

Foldvary N, Klem G, Hammel J, et al. The localizing value of ictal EEG in focal epilepsy. *Neurology* 2001;57:2022–2028.

Pacia SV, Ebersole JS. Intracranial EEG substsrates of scalp ictal patterns from temporal lobe foci. *Epilepsia* 1997;38:642–654.

So, EL. Value and limitations of seizure semiology in localizing seizure onset. *J Clin Neurophysiol* 2006;23:353–357.

Tatum WO IV. Long-term EEG monitoring: a clinical approach to electrophysiology. *J Clin Neurophysiol* 2001;18(5):442–455.

Verma A, Radtke R. EEG of partial seizures. *J Clin Neurophysiol* 2006;23: 333–339.

Westmoreland BF. The EEG findings in extratemporal seizures. *Epilepsia* 1998;39(Suppl 4):S1–S8.

Patterns of Special Significance

WILLIAM O. TATUM, IV

SELIM R. BENBADIS

AATIF M. HUSAIN

PETER W. KAPLAN

Many patterns of special significance are recorded in the intensive care unit (ICU) in patients that are critically ill with or without seizures. Nonepileptic encephalopathic recordings as well as those that are epileptiform occur in addition to those that include both forms with dynamic transition. In stupor and coma, slower waveforms are seen that are morphologically different than those that are seen during sleep. With greater depths of coma, EEG typically reflects a greater degree of worsening, although progression is different in different individuals and most patterns are nonspecific. However, some patterns have special prognostic significance and will be represented in the following section. The interictal-ictal continuum has been best elucidated in the study of status epilepticus (SE). This chapter will serve as a supplement to previous topics (see Chapters 2–4). Patterns of severe encephalopathies often associated with stupor or coma as well as SE will be illustrated. In coma, EEG may be useful to quantify the degree of cerebral dysfunction, help localize an abnormality, or assist with etiology in addition to noninvasively following clinical or response to treatment. While many encephalopathic forms of special significance are infrequently seen, SE is common and deserves special mention.

The diagnosis of SE has largely been clinical, particularly with convulsive status epilepticus (CSE). The EEG has shown great promise with the advent of long term monitoring (LTM) in cases with impaired consciousness. Frequently, readily identifiable clinical features are less apparent to observers, thus increasing the importance of EEG in the ongoing management of the stuporous or comatose patient in intensive care settings. Nonconvulsive events such as eye blinking and deviation, nystagmus, face and limb myoclonus, staring, or subtle mental status changes depend on the use of EEG in diagnosing and classifying these as nonconvulsive SE. No particular EEG pattern is representative for the clinical type of seizure or SE depicting it as convulsive or nonconvulsive. SE represents the temporal extension of individual seizures, and therefore the type of SE reflects the various types of epileptic seizures with their different EEG patterns. Similar to the seizure types previously demonstrated in Chapter 4, the EEG classification of SE can be divided into generalized and focal patterns. Intermediate examples may occur, with the evolution of a focal to a generalized pattern, or the reverse. This spread of seizure activity may exhibit an evolution in spatial spread, discharge amplitude, and frequency throughout the course of SE. Between individual discharges, there may be preservation (or conversely ablation) of background activity. Patterns may exhibit continuous or discontinuous features. Periodic discharges (PDs) may be seen focally or bilaterally in a variety of patterns associated with seizures and SE. When PDs are present, they may appear synchronous, or have independent hemispheric periodicity. The EEG of SE typically contains individual discharges. These may wax and wane and occur in a frequency of less than every several seconds to >3/sec. They may contain spike, sharp wave, polyspike morphologies, or mixtures of these features. The morphologies may occur focally, regionally, or in a generalized distribution.

PERIODIC EPILEPTIFORM DISCHARGES

Periodic patterns are characterized by repetitive waveforms that often appear as being epileptiform and recur in a persistent, regular, and periodic (or pseudoperiodic) fashion. The etiology for periodic patterns is nonspecific, although, when identified bilaterally, they usually reflect an acute or subacute, diffuse, encephalopathic process. When identified unilaterally, they often reflect a focal structural manifestation when lateralized and persistent. Some of the periodic patterns (periodic lateralized epileptiform discharges [PLEDs], bilateral PLEDs [BiPLEDs], generalized periodic epileptiform discharges [GPEDs]) may appear in patients with stupor and coma. Morphology, field of involvement, and reactivity are important in quantifying the patterns within the context of the state of consciousness. Discharges that repeat at regular intervals are periodic or pseudoperiodic and may reflect the continuum of epileptiform abnormality or epileptic encephalopathies that have the potential for manifesting seizures. These patterns may suggest more specific diagnoses when the patterns on EEG have characteristic features. The addition of movement monitors may help document a relationship in individuals between a periodic pattern and a clinical manifestation such as myoclonic jerks.

An interictal-ictal transition is represented within an indistinct spectrum of electrographic findings that may often times overlap (i.e., PLEDs). An electrographic seizure is not simply the repetition of interictal epileptiform discharges (IEDs) as is the case with the 3-Hz spike-and- wave pattern associated with idiopathic generalized epilepsy. Neither is it typically the prolongation of an interictal discharge, such as a polyspike, as in the case of generalized paroxysmal fast activity (GPFA) in patients with tonic seizures and symptomatic generalized epilepsy.

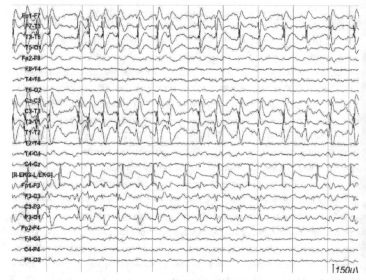

FIGURE 5.1. Frequent asymptomatic left temporal spike-and-slow waves in localization-related epilepsy (LRE).

When IEDs repeat themselves, symptoms may or may not arise, and repetitive IEDs are an infrequent ictal pattern as seen on EEG during seizures. Above is an individual with epilepsy who is asymptomatic at the time of the EEG recording despite the almost continuous repetitive IEDs (see Chapter 4 for similar features with symptoms).

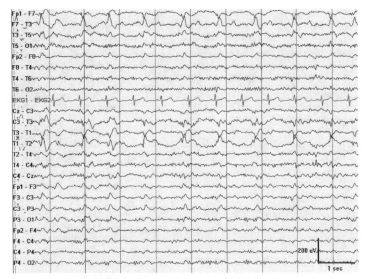

FIGURE 5.2. Left temporal PLEDs in a patient with left temporal lobe epilepsy immediately following serial complex partial seizure.

Periodic lateralized epileptiform discharges (PLEDs) are characteristically seen in acute (or subacute), pathological processes associated with a unilateral hemispheric structural lesion. However, PLEDs may appear as a physiological condition exacerbated by chronic conditions such as following seizures or rarely migraine. This periodic pattern is usually transient, typically disappearing in weeks. PLEDs are an interictal phenomenon, although they may be ictal when frequent and/or associated with rhythmic ictal discharges (see below). Partial-onset seizures occur in >70% of patients with PLEDs during their course.

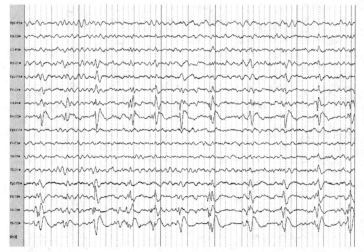

FIGURE 5.3. Left temporal PLEDs plus in a patient with an acute occipital ischemic infarction. Note the rhythmic ictal discharge abutting the discharge.

PLEDs plus may occur in the form of spikes, polyspikes, or sharp biphasic or triphasiform discharges with or without slow waves that repeat at regular periodic intervals. They typically appear in conjunction with an encephalopathy (with a diffusely slow background). Acute cerebral infarction or hemorrhage, tumors, anoxia, and central nervous system infections may evoke PLEDs, although they are nonspecific in etiology. Consciousness is impaired ranging from mild encephalopathy to coma. Status epilepticus is more commonly associated with PLEDs plus than with PLEDs (proper).

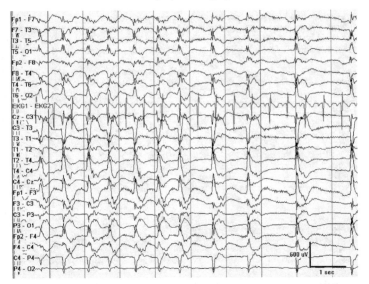

FIGURE 5.4. Generalized periodic epileptiform discharges. This ictal pattern followed a prolonged seizure. Note the high amplitude of the discharges.

Generalized periodic epileptiform discharges (GPEDs) are most often associated with encephalopathy (see above) and typically occur as an epiphenomena of a severe bilateral disturbance of cerebral dysfunction. However, GPEDs may appear as an ictal correlate when seizures are clinically evident. When GPEDs represent an ictal correlate, the state of the patient is less altered, a clinical presentation with seizures (not myoclonus) may be evident, and a visible background may be better visualized. See next section on stupor and coma.

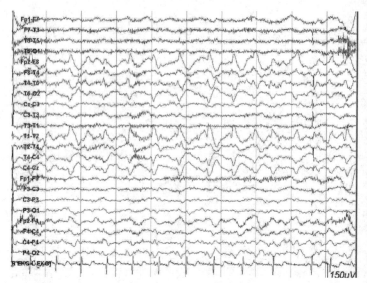

FIGURE 5.5. Right temporal PLEDs in a patient with herpes encephalitis and nonconvulsive SE recorded in the ICU.

The hallmark of herpes simplex encephalitis (HSE) is the presence of pseudoperiodic slow complexes or PLEDs in the setting of symptoms that suggest a central nervous system infectious disease. Initially a diffusely slow background is seen that within the first week manifests the periodic pattern. They are characteristically unilateral, but may be bilateral and independent and temporal in predominance. The discharges recur with a period of 1.0 to 2.5 sec and abate after weeks.

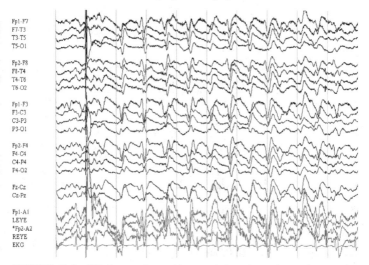

FIGURE 5.6. CJD in a patient with encephalopathy and myoclonic jerks. (Courtesy of Susan Herman, MD.)

Periodic discharges are the hallmark of Creutzfeldt-Jakob disease (CJD) and occur in the majority of patients. The pattern is a pseudoperiodic generalized sharp wave that occurs with a diffuse slow background. The discharges consist of biphasic or triphasic sharply contoured waveforms of varying durations that repeat with a period of 0.5 to 2.0 sec and shorten with disease progression. They are rarely unilateral, and appear within 3 months of onset in almost all patients. They are typically anterior predominant and are frequently time locked to myoclonic jerks.

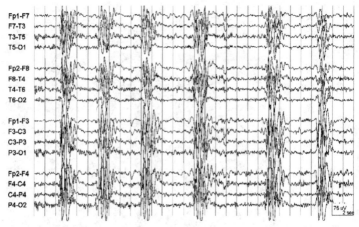

FIGURE 5.7. SSPE (early) in a patient presenting with encephalopathy and periodic episodes of atonia. (Courtesy of Susan Herman, MD.)

Subacute sclerosing panencephalitis (SSPE) is a chronic viral infection associated with measles that is now rare since the vaccine for measles prevention has become widespread. The EEG of SSPE has a characteristic pattern that is almost always present except in the very early phases of the disease. High voltage (>300 µV) slow waves or sharp-and-slow wave complexes lasting 0.5 to 2.0 sec repeat every 4 to 10 sec in a very regular pattern, and may be provoked by hyperventilation or sleep early in the course of the disease (see above). Discharges are diffuse, synchronous, and periodic or pseudoperiodic usually associated with slow myoclonic jerks or brief posturing.

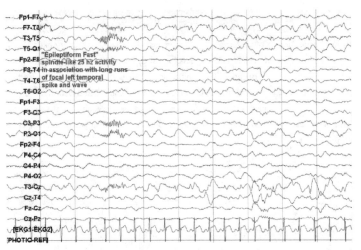

FIGURE 5.8. Nearly continuous left temporal-parietal seizures were found on EEG after magnetic resonance imaging (MRI) failed to demonstrate a lesion in a patient with abrupt onset of aphasia.

When patients with PLEDs on the EEG have seizures, they often have a clinical behavior during the seizure that reflects the site of seizure onset. While PLEDs proper reflect an epiphenomena typically of acute gray matter injury, focal rhythmic ictal fast activity associated with periodic complexes (seen above), short intervals of recurrence, and abnormal background between discharges are clues that the periodic complexes are more likely to represent an ictal phenomenon.

STUPOR AND COMA

A heightened index of suspicion for nonconvulsive seizures or status epilepticus is required when an individual with a neurological dysfunction develops an alteration of mental status. Prolonged EEG monitoring is increasingly becoming utilized to detect subtle or electrographic seizures that are not apparent in those that are clinically ill. The EEG is useful in demonstrating the degree of cerebral dysfunction but also with serial measurements in demonstrating dynamic changes that affect cerebral function.

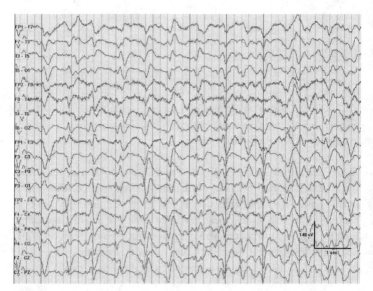

FIGURE 5.9. Diffuse slowing of the background rhythms with intermixed frontally predominant triphasic waves in a patient receiving hemodialysis in the critical care unit (CCU).

Triphasic waves are usually due to, but not limited to, encephalopathies associated with toxic and/or metabolic derangement that involve altered states of consciousness. The waveforms have three phases with a prominent high-voltage, surface-positive deflection sandwiched between a lower amplitude initial surface negative deflection and an aftergoing slower surface- negative potential. Triphasic waves are seen in bilateral nonevolving bursts or runs of 1 to 2 Hz frequently with an anterior predominance and an anterior to posterior lag, although they may also possess a posterior predominance, or mixed predominance. They may be reactive to eye opening or even benzodiazepine administration. When they occur in prolonged runs, distinguishing triphasic waves from nonconvulsive status epilepticus can be difficult.

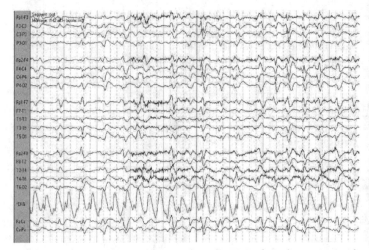

FIGURE 5.10. Triphasic waves noted on the EEG of another patient with encephalopathy due to renal failure, who is on hemodialysis. The EKG however, demonstrates ventricular fibrillation. The patient had a cardiac arrest and died during long-term EEG monitoring.

The electrocardiogram (EKG) is normally recorded on every EEG. Cardiac function has been inextricably related to brain function, and while many channels are dedicated to recording the EEG, the representation for cardiac function is based upon a single channel. The normal cardiac rhythm is usually represented by a bipolar derivation connecting the left to right chest. Various artifacts may appear in the EEG, although cardiac rhythm disturbances may be detected that are important for cerebral function or even predicate discovery of malignant arrhythmias (see above).

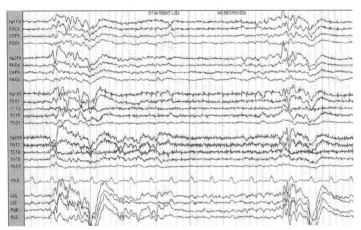

FIGURE 5.11. Burst-suppression following out-of-hospital cardiac arrest. The recording was obtained at 2 µV/mm with single electrode distances.

Burst suppression suggests a severe bilateral cerebral dysfunction, and while nonspecific in etiology, when associated with hypoxia, this pattern suggests a poor prognosis. The burst-suppression pattern consists of stereotyped bursts, usually consisting of mixed frequencies with or without intermixed epileptiform discharges. The bursts usually recur between 2 and 10 sec and are separated by intervals of suppression that demonstrate no electrocerebral activity at normal sensitivities. Note the lack of response to somatosensory stimulation annotated by the technologist.

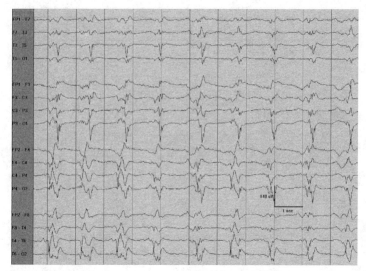

FIGURE 5.12. GPEDs in a 75-year-old man after cardiac arrest. He was comatose but had no clinical signs that were otherwise evident. Note the periodicity.

Generalized periodic epileptiform discharges (GPEDs) are bilateral periodic epileptiform discharges. They signify a diffuse encephalopathy and may occur with seizures, although frequently GPEDs occur as the expression of a diffuse structural injury pattern involving gray matter without seizures. They are unreactive to somatosensory stimulation, and are associated with an absent or diffusely slow posterior dominant rhythm. This pattern may also be seen with NCSE, and whether the EEG independent of overt seizures represents nonconvulsive SE often has been subject to clinical debate.

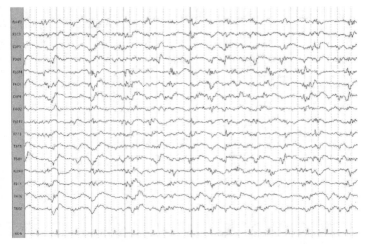

FIGURE 5.13. BiPLEDs in a 37-year-old HIV-positive man admitted following a prolonged generalized tonic-clonic seizure and meningoencephalitis. Note the right frontal and left occipital bilateral independent hemispheric discharges.

Bilateral independent periodic epileptiform discharges (BiPLEDs) are less commonly associated with seizures than are periodic lateralized epileptiform discharges (PLEDs). The discharges are bihemispheric and independent with different morphologies and periods of repetition and are less associated with seizures than are PLEDs or PLEDs plus. They are seen in patients with a severe bilateral disturbance of cerebral function, and while nonspecific, BiPLEDs are most commonly associated with hypoxic injury to the brain.

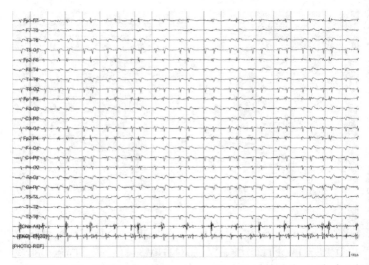

FIGURE 5.14. GPED suppression in anoxic encephalopathy with facial myoclonus reflected in the lower second chin electromyographic (EMG) channel. (Courtesy of Greg Fisher, MD.)

Generalized periodic epileptiform discharges (GPEDs) may be composed of spikes, polyspikes, or sharp waves that are bilateral and synchronous at a rate of 0.5 to 1.0 Hz on a "flat" or low-amplitude recording and be associated with frequent myoclonic jerks (status myoclonus). This pattern is seen with severe diffuse cerebral insults such as with massive hypoxia, typically after cardiac arrest, but also can be seen with stroke, trauma, or infections. The EEG typically lacks background activity between discharges and may reveal a burst-suppression pattern, GPEDs (see above), or prolonged periods of diffuse suppression. The outcome is characteristically grim, resulting in death or persistent vegetative states.

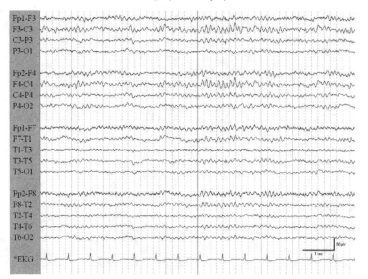

FIGURE 5.15. Alpha coma in a post–cardiopulmonary resusitation comatose patient following cardiac arrest. Stimulation was ineffective in creating a change in background.

Alpha coma is represented by diffuse alpha frequencies that are part of an unreactive pattern without anterior-posterior gradient on EEG seen in patients in coma. It is most frequently seen in hypoxic encephalopathy, although it has been reported with brainstem lesions, and portends a poor prognosis. Etiology is the most important determinant in outcome regardless of the patterns seen. Other coma patterns including beta coma, theta/delta coma, and spindle coma may also be seen. As with alpha coma, drugs and trauma carry a more favorable prognosis than hypoxic-ischemic causes.

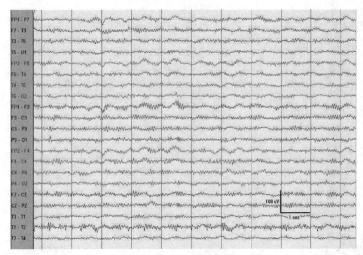

FIGURE 5.16. The EEG of a 67-year-old patient following cardiac arrest. Note the diffuse anterior predominant spindle-like activity.

Spindle coma is a pattern seen in comatose patients. Features on the EEG include prominent spindle-like activity similar to the spindles seen in stage 2 sleep, although they reflect abnormal spindle formation because they are unreactive, diffuse, and the patient is comatose. Etiologies are similar to alpha coma, with anoxia not being infrequently seen. It may also be seen with posttraumatic etiologies and, in this case, usually carries a better prognosis.

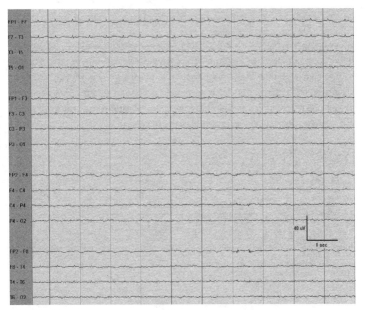

FIGURE 5.17. A 52-year-old following cardiac arrest 10 days previously. The patient met the clinical criteria for a diagnosis of brain death.

Electrocerebral inactivity is defined as no cerebral activity greater than 2 μV. For the purpose of brain death recording, guidelines produced by the American Clinical Neurophysiology Society (ACNS) are available and include several other requirements, such as testing the integrity of the system and recording at double interelectrode distances, and ensuring electrode impedances are between 100 and 5000 ohms. In addition, certain factors that may make this pattern reversible must be excluded, such as hypothermia and sedative drugs. EEG is considered an indirect and adjunct test for clinical brain death, but is not required for the diagnosis.

STATUS EPILEPTICUS

Status epilepticus represents prolonged seizures with various electroclinical patterns on EEG. All seizure types may manifest as status epilepticus. The features of status epilepticus seen on the EEG are a reflection of the seizure type with characteristic electrographic patterns. Both convulsive and nonconvulsive forms occur, and prolonged EEG recording can help elucidate the temporal pattern of patients with recurrent seizures when subtle or no clinical signs are present.

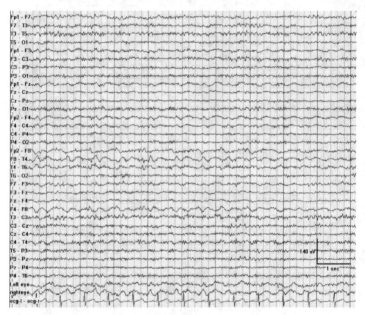

FIGURE 5.18. Epilepsia partialis continua in a 41-year-old patient with subjective tingling and "twitching" noted at the corner of the left side of the mouth. Note the rhythmic delta frequencies on the EEG that phase reverse at the F8 derivation.

The diagnosis of simple partial status epilepticus is confirmed by the presence of an electrographic correlate on EEG. This occurs in a minority of cases of suspected SPSE given the restricted epileptogenic zone that is involved. The discharges favor the convexity of the cerebral hemispheres, and hence EEG may reveal spikes over frontal, rolandic, parietal, or occipital regions. When temporal discharges are found and a clinical correlate is present, these regions beyond an experiential sensation usually are projected from extratemporal sources. Depending on the region involved, seizures may begin with polyspike activity, rhythmic activity or spike-slow-wave activity. When localized to a single restricted area, SPSE is referred to as *epilepsia partialis continua*.

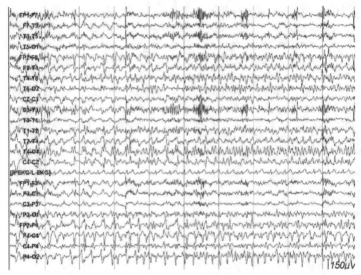

FIGURE 5.19. Complex partial SE in a 21-year-old patient with postencephalitic localization-related epilepsy. The clinical symptoms were mild confusion. Note the right hemispheric ictal activity.

Complex partial SE is often characterized by a change in mental status with impairment of consciousness. EEG patterns may include repetitive spiking, spike-slow-wave, rhythmic low- voltage fast activity, or a combination of sharps and slow frequencies. The patterns may wax and wane showing changes in frequency and amplitude as well as in spatial distribution (see above). Although seizures are usually seen unilaterally, they may be seen bilaterally, independently, or may propagate from one hemisphere to the other. Complex partial SE may initially lateralize with 4-to 7-Hz rhythmic activity during clinical symptomatology. When the convexity of the temporal lobe is the origin, the EEG shows more widely distributed rhythmic activity.

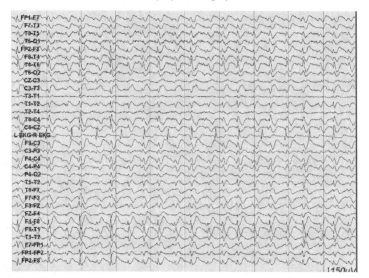

FIGURE 5.20. EEG in a patient with postanoxic generalized nonconvulsive SE that followed convulsive SE.

Electrographic seizures seen during EEG may be found during the evaluation of comatose patients. They can occur after convulsive status epilepticus, or be uncovered in comatose patients with few clinical clues other than a change in mental status. The EEG may show generalized periodic discharges, polyspikes, spike-and-slow-waves or even diffuse, rhythmic waxing and waning delta or theta activity. The EEG may appear focal or diffuse and have IEDs that are serial or continuous as with nonconvulsive status epilepticus (NCSE). Note the generalized spike-wave complexes with right lateralization in the above example. There are a wide variety of possible EEG patterns that may be seen with NCSE.

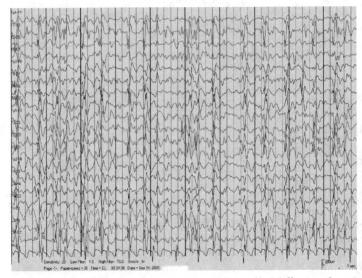

FIGURE 5.21. ESES in a 9-year-old boy with Landau-Kleffner syndrome. No clinical features were noted.

Landau-Kleffner syndrome (LKS) and the syndrome of continuous spikes and waves during slow sleep (CSWS) are syndromes of acquired language (LKS) or cognitive dysfunction (CSWS) associated with seizures in about three-fourths of patients. Irrespective of seizures, consistent IEDs appear while awake, although in varying degrees and locations. They may be high-voltage multifocal spikes and spike-wave discharges that occur singly or in salvos, unilaterally or bilaterally, and often involving the posterior temporal (language dominant) head regions. The IEDs during slow-wave sleep appear diffuse, symmetrical, or asymmetrical bisynchronous, and increase so that 85% of the recording or more comprises electrical status epilepticus of slow sleep (ESES).

ADDITIONAL RESOURCES

American Clinical Neurophysiology Society. Guideline 3: Minimum technical standards for EEG recording in suspected cerebral death. *J Clin Neurophysiol* 2006;23:97–104.

Boulanger JM, Deacon C, Lecuyer D, et al. Triphasic waves versus nonconvulsive status epilepticus: EEG distinction. *Can J Neurol Sci* 2006;33:175–180.

Brenner RP, Schaul N. Periodic EEG patterns: classification, clinical correlation, and pathophysiology. *J Clin Neurophysiol* 1990;7:249–267.

Herman ST. In: FW Drislane, ed. *Status Epilepticus*. Humana Press, Totowa, NJ, 2005:245–262.

Kaplan PW. Non-convulsive status epilepticus. *Semin Neurol* 1996;16:33–40.

Kaplan PW. The EEG of status epilepticus. *J Clin Neurophysiol.* 2006;23:221–229.

Kaplan PW, Genoud D, Ho TW, Jallon P. Etiology, neurologic correlations, and prognosis in alpha coma. *Clin Neurophysiol* 1999;110:205–213.

Kaplan PW, Genoud D, Ho TW, Jallon P. Clinical correlates and prognosis in early spindle coma. *Clin Neurophysiol* 2000;111:584–90.

Shorvon S, Walker M. Status epilepticus in idiopathic generalized epilepsies. *Epilepsia* 2005; 46:73–79.

Tatum WO, French JA, Benbadis SR, Kaplan PW. The etiology and diagnosis of status epilepticus. *Epilep Behav* 2001;2:311–317.

Treiman DM. Electroclinical features of status epilepticus. *J Clin Neurophysiol.* 1995;12:343–362.

Polysomnography

AATIF M. HUSAIN

S leep is a nonhomogenous state composed of mostly non–rapid eye movement (NREM) and rapid eye movement (REM) sleep. NREM sleep is further divided into four stages, starting with light sleep (stage I) to deep sleep (stage IV). Sleep and its disorders are often studied with a polysomnogram (PSG), also known as a sleep study. A PSG allows one to determine the quantity and quality of sleep.

The terms listed below are commonly used in PSG

1. Lights out: start of PSG
2. Lights on: end of PSG
3. TIB (time in bed): total time patient was in bed during sleep study (including periods of wakefulness)
4. TST (total sleep time): total time patient was in bed in any stage of sleep
5. Sleep efficiency: (TST/TIB) × 100, expressed as percentage
6. WASO (wakefulness after sleep onset): time spent awake after the first epoch of sleep and before final awakening
7. Sleep latency: time from lights out to first stage of sleep
8. REM latency: time from first stage of sleep to first epoch of REM sleep
9. % Stages I, II, III, IV, REM: (time spent in each stage/TST) × 100, expressed as percentage; often stages III and IV are expressed together as slow-wave (or delta) sleep.

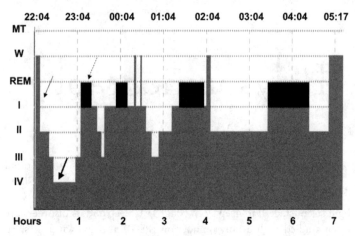

FIGURE 6.1. Hypnogram of normal sleep cycle.

The hypnogram is a graphic representation of sleep stages achieved in an overnight polysomnogram. The features noted in Figure 6.1 reflect the normal sleep cycle in a single overnight recording for an adult. Non-REM sleep consists of light sleep (stages I and II, *thin arrow*) and deep sleep (stages III and IV, *dashed arrow*) repeating four to five times per night. REM, or "dream sleep," occurs throughout the night, appearing approximately every 90 min.

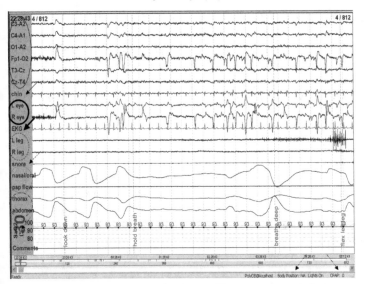

FIGURE 6.2. A 30-sec page (epoch) of a PSG demonstrating a typical montage.

In a routine PSG, many physiological parameters are recorded to determine the normal and abnormal features or stages of sleep. Physiological parameters commonly recorded are included in Figure 6.2; electroencephalogram (EEG) (*thin oval*), chin electromyogram (EMG) (*thin arrow*), eye movements (electro-oculogram, EOG) (*thick circle*), electrocardiogram (ECG) (*thick arrow*), leg movements (leg EMG) (*dashed circle*), snoring (*dashed arrow*), airflow (*dotted circle*), respiratory effort (*dashed-dotted circle*), and oxygen saturation. Additionally, body position (*dashed-dotted arrow*), oxygen supplementation, and continuous positive airway pressure (CPAP) are also noted (*dashed-dotted-dotted arrow*). Initial PSGs used a single EEG channel, C3-A2 or C4-A1, to score sleep stages. Later, however, at least one other channel using an occipital electrode (O1 or O2) was added to aid in determining transition to sleep. In patients in whom epileptic seizures are in the differential diagnosis, a full set of EEG electrodes is applied and 16 to 18 channels of EEG are recorded. This allows a more definitive diagnosis of interictal and ictal epileptiform abnormalities. Chin EMG is recorded from the submental region. This helps in staging of sleep, with highest chin EMG activity noted in wakefulness and lowest in REM sleep. Some sleep disorders cause characteristic EMG abnormalities, such as increased tonic and phasic EMG activity during REM sleep. EOG leads are placed below the outer canthus of the left eye and above the outer canthus of the right eye. Thus, any deflection of the eyes, whether horizontal or vertical, produces an out of phase deflection. ECG monitoring electrodes are placed on the anterior chest wall. This is used to detect cardiac arrhythmias in sleep; it is not adequate for assessment of subtle abnormalities of cardiac conduction. Leg leads are used to monitor EMG activity (movements) in the legs. Electrodes are placed on the anterior tibialis muscle bilaterally. Dorsiflexion of the great toe and foot is monitored with these electrodes. Respiratory monitoring involves assessment of airflow, respiratory effort, and oxygen saturation. At times, a snore microphone is also used to detect snoring. Airflow is monitored with nasal and oral thermistors or pressure transducers. Ventilatory effort is measured by recording chest and abdominal movements. Pulse oximetry is used to determine oxygen saturation. Other pertinent information, such as the patient's position, whether they are using supplemental oxygen, and CPAP, if it is being used, is also noted. It is standard to review PSG in 30- sec intervals (pages or epochs), which is equivalent to a display speed of 10 mm/sec. Each epoch is scored according to the prevailing sleep stage. At the start of every PSG, the technologist asks the patient to perform various tasks, such as eye blinks, breath holding, moving legs, and others, to test the integrity of the system and to make sure that appropriate deflections are noted.

NORMAL SLEEP

Normally, sleep cycles remain consistent throughout the life of an individual and throughout development and aging. Overnight polygraphic recordings include EEG and other measures of ventilation, airflow, cardiac function, and muscle movements. Polysomnograms are the foundation for assessing the normalcy of sleep architecture, respiration, and nocturnal behavioral events. Multiple sleep latency or wakefulness testing is another technique to determine the latency of sleep onset or REM onset.

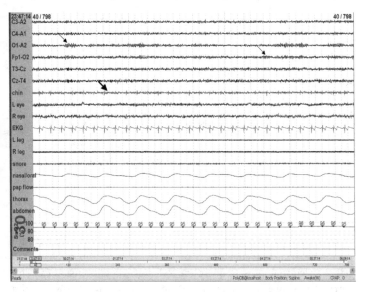

FIGURE 6.3. This is a 30-sec epoch demonstrating stage W with alpha activity in the occipital channels (*thin arrows*) and tonic EMG activity (*thick arrow*).

Stage W, or normal wakefulness, is often seen at the start of a PSG and after awakenings. Characteristic features include alpha rhythm in the occipital regions, tonic EMG, rapid eye blinks, and regular respiration. Occasionally, instead of an alpha rhythm, low-voltage, mixed-frequency activity is seen.

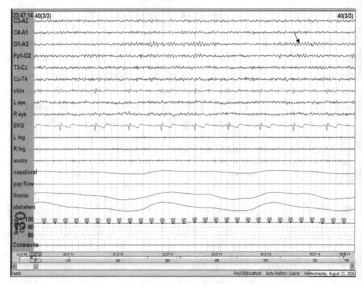

FIGURE 6.4. This is a 10-sec epoch of stage W; it is the last 10 sec of the previous sample.

This sample is displayed at the same paper speed (30 mm/sec) as used in routine EEG. The alpha activity in the occipital electrodes looks similar to that seen in a routine EEG (*arrow*); in this case, it is occurring at a frequency of about 11 Hz. It is helpful to change the paper speed to a more familiar one to better recognize usual EEG features. The slower paper speed (10 mm/sec) used in PSG is useful as low-frequency activity (such as respiration) is better seen at that paper speed.

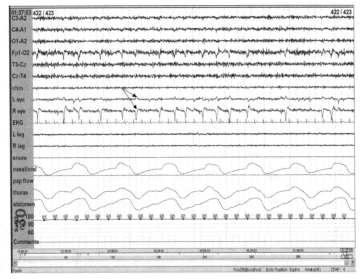

FIGURE 6.5. This is a 30-sec epoch of stage W with frequent eye blinks present (*arrows*).

This sample has an alpha rhythm in the occipital region, tonic EMG, and regular respiration. In addition, frequent eye blinks are also seen. Eye blinks appear as out of phase deflections in the eye leads. Along with alpha rhythm, tonic EMG, and regular respiration, eye blinks are frequently seen in stage W.

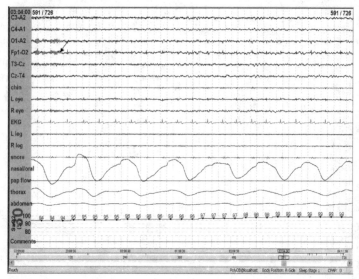

FIGURE 6.6. This is a 30-sec epoch showing sleep onset at about the third second (*arrow*).

The initial change in EEG between stage W and stage I is fragmentation of the alpha activity. Occipital electrodes are more sensitive in recording alpha activity fragmentation. As seen in this tracing, the first sign of sleep onset is loss of alpha activity (*arrow*) best seen in the O1-A2 and Fp1-O2 channels. At the same time, no significant change occurs in the C3-A2 channel. Consequently, contemporary PSG always include at least two EEG channels: C3-A2 or C4-A1 and O1-A2 or O2-A1. Many laboratory use additional channels to aid further with sleep staging.

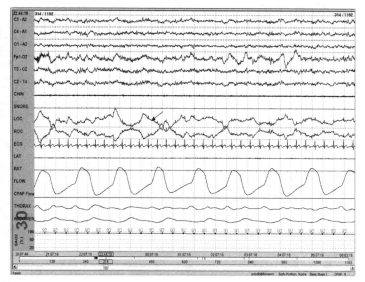

FIGURE 6.7. This is a 30-sec epoch demonstrating early stage I sleep with slow rolling eye movements (*arrow*).

Stage I sleep is the transitional phase seen between wakefulness and deeper stages of sleep. It comprises mostly a mixed-frequency activity in the 2- to 7-Hz range. Early in stage I sleep, the alpha rhythm becomes fragmented to a slower frequency activity and slow rolling eye movements appear. Slow eye movements are distinguished from rapid eye movements by the duration of the up slope of the eye movement; rapid eye movements have an up slope of less than 300 msec, whereas the up slope of slow eye movements is greater than 500 msec. EMG activity in this stage of sleep is less than in wakefulness, but greater than in deeper stages of sleep. Later in stage I sleep, vertex sharp waves appear, but K complexes and sleep spindles are not present.

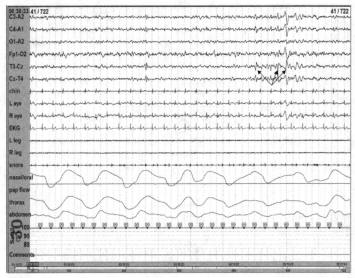

FIGURE 6.8. This is a 30-sec epoch showing late stage I sleep.

In this epoch of stage I sleep, the EEG consists of mixed-frequency activity, mostly in the 2- to 7-Hz range, and the slow eye movements have disappeared. Vertex potentials, which are present in the later stages of stage I sleep, are seen (*arrows*). As their name implies, vertex potentials are surface-negative waves that phase reverse over the vertex (Cz). At times, they can be of high amplitude, reaching 200 µV.

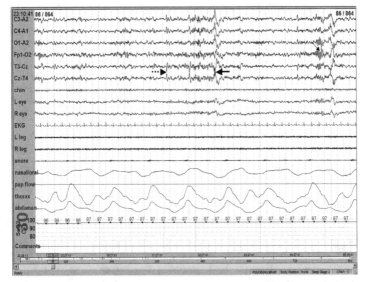

FIGURE 6.9. This is a 30-sec epoch demonstrating stage II sleep with vertex waves (*dashed arrow*), sleep spindles (*thin arrow*), and K complexes (*thick arrow*).

Stage II sleep can be scored only if sleep spindles or K complexes are present. Sleep spindles consist of 11- to 14-Hz waves that must last at least 0.5 sec. K complexes have an initial negative sharp wave followed by a positive component. They are seen maximally over the vertex (Cz). In scoring stage II sleep, sleep spindles and K complexes are transient discharges and may not be seen in every epoch. As long as successive sleep spindles or K complexes are seen less than 3 min apart, the intervening sleep is scored as stage II. Otherwise, the intervening sleep is scored as stage I if the architecture of other sleep stages is not present. The EMG in stage II sleep is less than in stage I but more than that seen in deeper stages of sleep.

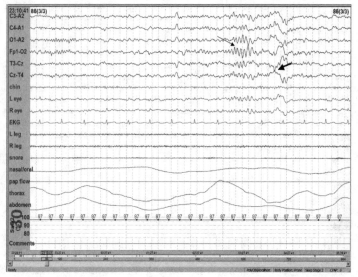

FIGURE 6.10. This is a 10-sec epoch of stage II; it is the last 10 sec of the previous sample.

This sample is displayed at the same time base (30 mm/sec) as used in routine EEG. The 11- Hz activity lasting for over 1 sec is a sleep spindle (*thin arrow*), whereas a K complex is seen 1 sec later (*thick arrow*). As with other types of sleep architecture, it is often useful to change the paper speed from 10 mm/sec to 30 mm/sec for better identification of sleep spindles.

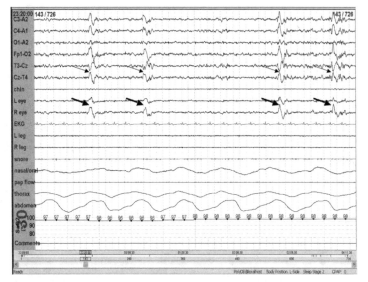

FIGURE 6.11. This is a 30-sec epoch demonstrating stage II sleep with recurrent K complexes.

Several K complexes can occur in a single epoch (*thin arrows*). K complexes often occur in response to a stimulus, but can occur spontaneously as well. At times, K complexes can be seen in the eye leads as well (*thick arrows*). This is easily differentiated from eye movements, as the latter have out of phase deflections as long as the eye leads are positioned above and below the outer canthus. The definitions of K complexes vary in PSG and EEG. In PSG, a K complex is defined as a biphasic wave with the maximum amplitude over the vertex and a duration of at least 0.5 sec. In EEG, a K complex does not have a duration criteria, but is defined as a biphasic wave with maximum amplitude over the vertex followed by a sleep spindle.

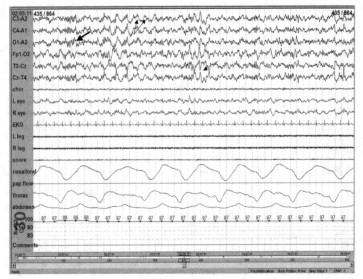

FIGURE 6.12. This is a 30-sec epoch demonstrating stage III sleep with slow waves present (*thin arrows*) that do not encompass more than 50% of the epoch. Additionally, sleep spindles are noted (*thick arrow*) as are vertex waves (*dashed arrow*).

Stage III sleep is scored when the EEG has high-amplitude slow waves occupying at least 20% but no more than 50% of the epoch. Slow waves are 2 Hz or slower and must have a peak to peak amplitude of at least 75 µV. Sleep spindles, K complexes, and vertex waves may or may not be present in this stage of sleep.

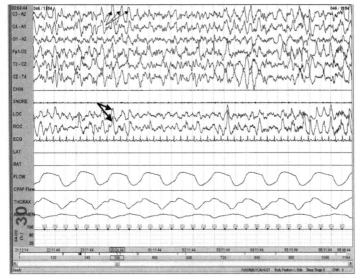

FIGURE 6.13. This is a 30-sec epoch demonstrating stage IV sleep and high-amplitude delta waves (*thin arrows*) that are often seen in the eye leads as well (*thick arrows*).

In stage IV sleep, slow waves encompass at least 50% of the epoch. Slow waves are defined the same way as in stage III sleep. Sleep spindles, K complexes, and vertex waves may or may not be present in stage IV sleep. Many PSG laboratories score stages III and IV together, as differentiation between the two stages is difficult, and is referred to as stage delta, delta sleep, or slow- wave sleep. Most of the delta waves above are greater than 100 µV. Delta waves can be differentiated from eye movements because these waves are in phase, and eye movements are out of phase in the eye leads. EMG activity is low in delta sleep; however not as low as in REM sleep.

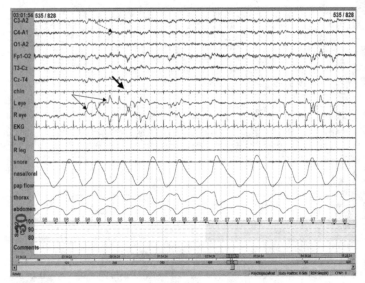

FIGURE 6.14. This is a 30-sec epoch demonstrating stage REM with frequent rapid eye movements (*thin arrows*), atonia (*thick arrow*), and mixed-frequency EEG (*dashed arrow*).

Stage REM is characterized by the appearance of low-amplitude, mixed-frequency EEG activity, EMG atonia, and rapid eye movements. EEG activity is similar to that seen in stage I sleep; however, vertex waves are much less common. Although EMG atonia is characteristic in stage REM, occasional phasic EMG bursts may be seen. If EMG atonia is not noted, the EMG must be at the lowest level compared to other stages of sleep (relative atonia). The most characteristic feature of this stage of sleep is the rapid eye movements, and can be distinguished from slow rolling eye movements by the rapid up slope of the eye movement. It is less than 300 msec in rapid eye movements. Note that the eye movements are seen as out of phase deflections in the eye leads, clearly differentiating them from brain activity. It is not unusual to see irregularity of respiration and cardiac rhythm in stage REM.

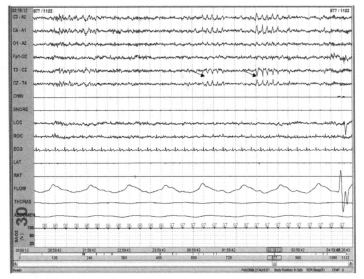

FIGURE 6.15. This is a 30-sec epoch showing the start of stage REM and saw tooth waves.

Saw tooth waves (*arrows*) are 2- to 5-Hz vertex negative sharp waves that often occur in a series. They can be precursors of stage REM or can occur with phasic bursts of EMG activity or rapid eye movements during stage REM. Rules for scoring the start and end of stage REM are complex, and the reader is referred to other comprehensive reviews.

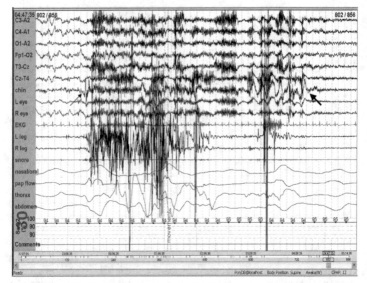

FIGURE 6.16. This is a 30-sec epoch that is scored as movement time. The movement starts at about second 5 (*thin arrow*) and ends at about the 25th second (*thick arrow*).

When at least 50% of an epoch contains movement artifact obscuring underlying EEG, EOG, and EMG, and it is preceded and followed by sleep, it is scored as movement time. This differentiates movement time from movements occurring during wakefulness. Also, shorter duration movements (obscuring less than 50% of the epoch) are not scored as movement time but rather are scored according to the prevailing sleep stage. During this period, the underlying EEG cannot be accurately staged, and so this epoch is scored as movement time.

RESPIRATORY ABNORMALITIES

Respiratory abnormalities are often seen in patients with clinical complaints of excessive daytime sleepiness. Abnormalities of respiration are commonly encountered in sleep disorders. Apnea and hypopneas are abnormal periods of respiratory interruption that are frequently encountered in the diagnosis of sleep disorders.

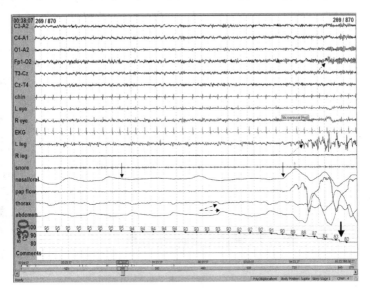

FIGURE 6.17. This is a 30-sec epoch demonstrating an obstructive apnea marked by *thin arrows* (about 16 sec). Note the desaturation at the end of the page that is occurring in response to the apnea (*thick arrow*) with an arousal (*dashed arrow*) and body movement (*dotted arrow*). Excursions of the thoracic and abdominal respiratory effort monitors demonstrate paradoxical respiration (*line and dash arrows*).

Although scoring rules for apneas differ, they must have a duration of at least 10 sec and airflow must be diminished by at least 90% compared to the airflow before and after the apnea. During this period of airflow cessation due to airway collapse, respiratory effort is manifested by ongoing excursions of the thoracic and abdominal belts. Instead of thoracic and abdominal movements being in phase as they normally are, in an apnea, they are out of phase. This is referred to as paradoxical respiration. After an apnea oxygen desaturation may result, and typically follows the apneas by 10 to 20 sec necessary to manifest the hypoxemia. At the termination of the apnea, there is usually a large breath, a body movement, and often an arousal.

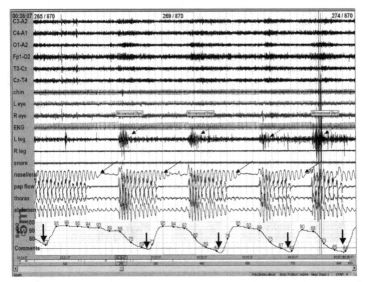

FIGURE 6.18. This is a 5-min epoch demonstrating frequent obstructive sleep apneas.

When evaluating respiration, it is helpful to use a long time base since the deflections of interest are very slow waves. The above sample is from the same patient as the prior sample. The long time base makes identification of respiratory dysrhythmias easy (*thin arrows*). Note also that following each apnea, there is a significant oxygen desaturation (*thick arrow*). A leg movement is also noted after every apnea as well (*dashed arrows*). Interpreting the EEG with such a long time base is difficult.

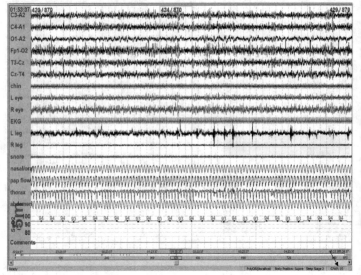

FIGURE 6.19. This is a 5-min epoch demonstrating of a patient with severe obstructive sleep apnea (OSA) that is being treated with CPAP.

Continuous positive airway pressure (CPAP) is an effective treatment for OSA. This epoch is from the same patient as the preceding two epochs. There is resolution of the apneas and desaturations with treatment with CPAP at a pressure of 10 cm H_2O (*arrow*).

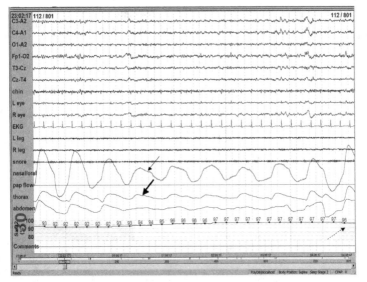

FIGURE 6.20. This is a 30-sec epoch demonstrating a 15-sec obstructive hypopnea. There is a 60% amplitude reduction in the nasal/oral airflow channel (*thin arrow*) with continued respiratory effort (*thick arrow*), and oxygen desaturation >4% that follows the event (overlaps to the next page [not shown]) (*dashed arrow*). The reduced airflow and oxygen desaturation allow this event to be scored as hypopnea.

Hypopnea scoring also may differ. Many laboratories use a greater than 50% but less than a 90% decrease in amplitude of the nasal/oral airflow channel that lasts for at least 10 sec, accompanied by an oxygen desaturation of at least 3% to 4% or an arousal. Apneas do not have the same requirement of being associated with either a desaturation or arousal. The physiological consequences of both obstructive apneas and hypopneas are the same; therefore, it has been recommended that these events not be scored separately. The term obstructive apnea/hypopnea event is used when there is a greater than 50% decrease of the amplitude of the nasal/oral airflow channel, or if the decrease is less than 50%, but is associated with at least a 3% desaturation or arousal. Like most definitions, the event must last at least 10 sec.

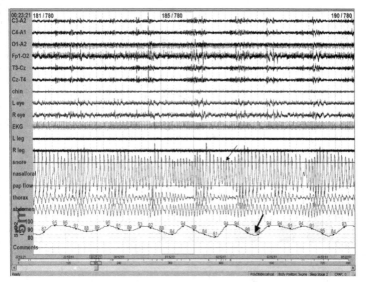

FIGURE 6.21. This is a 5-min epoch demonstrating obstructive hypopneas (*thin arrow*) associated with oxygen desaturations (*thick arrow*).

The American Academy of Sleep Medicine (AASM) recommends that obstructive apneas and hypopneas be counted as a single obstructive apnea/hypopnea event as their physiological consequences are similar. The epoch above illustrates the severity of hypopneas (approximately 50% reduction of the nasal/oral airflow channel), with a considerable desaturation (to about 80%) during each event.

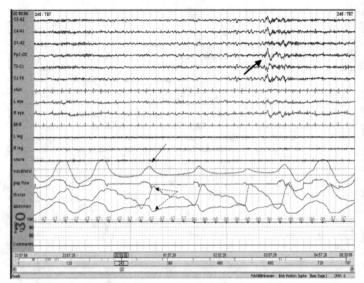

FIGURE 6.22. This is a 30-sec epoch demonstrating an obstructive hypopnea lasting 15 sec (*thin arrow*) and a subsequent arousal (*thick arrow*). Note the paradoxical respiration manifest in the respiratory effort monitors (*dashed arrows*).

Obstructive apneas and hypopneas are frequently associated with arousals. The degree of daytime sleepiness in obstructive sleep apnea correlates more with the number of arousal than with severity of apneas or desaturations. The arousal is manifest by an abrupt EEG frequency shift that lasts more than 3 sec.

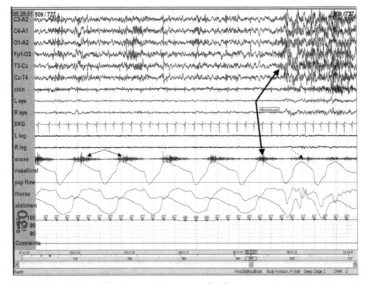

FIGURE 6.23. This is a 30-sec epoch demonstrating a respiratory event–related arousal. In this example, there is recurrent snoring (*thin arrows*) with one of the snores associated with an arousal (*thick arrow*). Notice how the snores diminish after the arousal (*dashed arrow*).

Periodically, patients have abnormal respiratory events that do not meet the scoring criteria for apneas and hypopneas but appear to be caused by airway compromise. These patients have loud snoring which is frequently associated with arousals. The AASM recommends that these events be called respiratory event related arousals (RERAs). Studies using esophageal pressure manometry show that these events are associated with an increase in negative intrapleural pressure similar to that seen in apneas and hypopneas. The AASM suggests that these events be counted with obstructive apnea/hypopnea events. RERAs often resolve with CPAP.

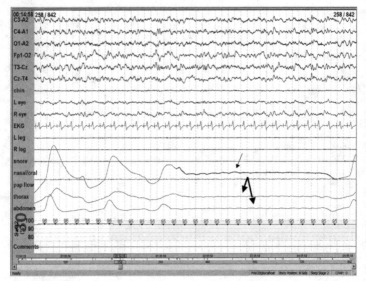

FIGURE 6.24. This is a 30-sec epoch demonstrating a central apnea with absence of both nasal/oral airflow (*thin arrow*) and respiratory effort (*thick arrows*).

In central apnea, there is not only cessation of airflow but also of respiratory effort, as noted by the thoracic and abdominal channels. In some patients, weak respiratory efforts may go undetected by the thoracic and abdominal channels, or an obstructive apnea may mimic a central one. Central apneas can occur in neuromuscular disorders, neurological disorders involving primarily the brain stem, heart failure, high altitudes, or they may be idiopathic.

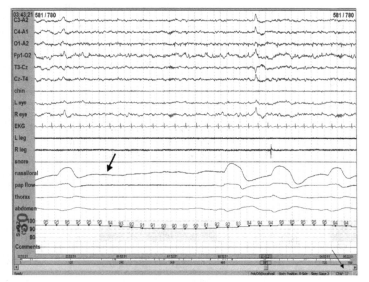

FIGURE 6.25. This is a 30-sec epoch demonstrating a central apnea in a patient undergoing CPAP titration for obstructive sleep apnea syndrome.

Central apneas can occur when patients with obstructive sleep apnea are undergoing CPAP titration. This pattern has recently been termed complex sleep apnea. If the CPAP pressure is increased beyond what is optimal for the patient, central apneas can occur. The patient in the sample above was previously diagnosed with obstructive sleep apnea and was undergoing this study for CPAP titration. The patient's obstructive events were eliminated at a CPAP pressure of 14 cm H_2O. The technologist continued to increase the CPAP pressure for occasional arousals, and at a pressure of 17 cm H_2O (*thin arrow*), the patient started to have central apneas (*thick arrow*). The optimal CPAP setting was for 14 cm H_2O. New BiPAP machines that may specifically treat this type of pattern have become available.

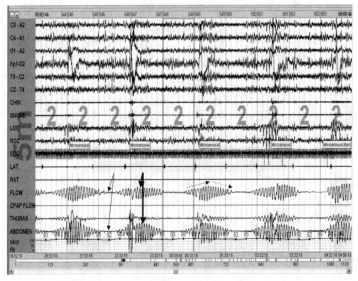

FIGURE 6.26. This is a 5-min epoch demonstrating Cheyne-Stokes respiration with periods of central apnea manifest by absence of nasal/oral airflow and respiratory effort (*thin arrows*), alternating with periods of hyperpnea (*thick arrows*).

Cheyne-Stokes respiration is a cyclical pattern in which there is waxing and waning of breathing between central apneas and periods of hyperpnea. This is usually seen in patients with congestive heart failure and cerebrovascular disease. The apneas may be associated with arousals or desaturations. Following an obstructive event, the apnea often result in a deep, high-amplitude breath. In Cheyne-Stokes respiration, there is gradual waxing of respiration after the apnea (*dashed arrow*). After the hyperpnea reaches its peak, the breathing starts waning again (*dotted arrow*).

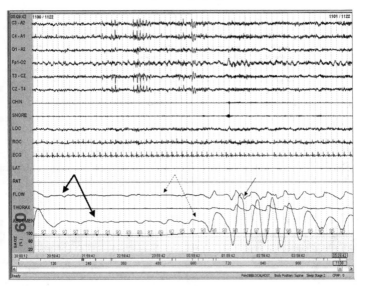

FIGURE 6.27. This is a 60-sec epoch that demonstrates a mixed apnea with the entire event and the compensatory breaths that terminate the event (*thin arrow*). Notice the initial part of the event in which there is a cessation of both nasal/oral airflow and respiratory effort (*thick arrow*).

Mixed apneas are considered a variant of obstructive apneas. During the first half of the event, respiratory effort appears to be absent, but is present in the latter half. Physiologically, mixed apneas are thought to have the same consequences as obstructive ones, and they are often counted together. The AASM also encourages counting them with obstructive apnea/hypopnea events. In the latter part of the event, there continues to be cessation of nasal/oral airflow but respiratory effort returns (*dashed arrows*).

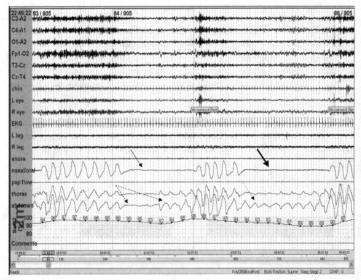

FIGURE 6.28. This is a 2-min epoch demonstrating both a mixed (*thin arrow*) and obstructive apnea (*thick arrow*).

As noted before, mixed apneas have the same physiological consequences as obstructive apneas. They often occur in the same patient, and both resolve with CPAP. Mixed and obstructive apneas can occur back to back in the same patient, suggesting that indeed they have a similar pathophysiology. Notice the absence of respiratory effort in the first half of the mixed apnea with return in the second half (*dashed arrows*). The obstructive apnea has persistence of respiratory effort from the beginning (*dotted arrow*).

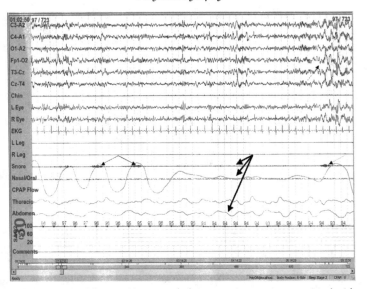

FIGURE 6.29. This is a 30-sec epoch demonstrating snoring associated with an obstructive apnea. Note that snoring occurs with every breath (*arrows*) typically at the peak of inspiration (*line*). In this patient, snoring is not associated with apneas, hypopneas, desaturations, or arousals.

In addition to monitoring nasal/oral airflow, respiratory effort, and oxygen saturation, many laboratories also record snoring with a small microphone attached to the side of the trachea. Snoring is often present with obstructive sleep apnea and represents subtle narrowing of the airway. In this sample, snoring is noted in the first third of the sample (*thin arrows*), but disappears during the obstructive apnea (*thick arrows*). At the termination of the apnea, there is an arousal (*dashed arrow*) and return of snoring (*dotted arrow*). During CPAP titration for this patient, an attempt should be made to eliminate not only the apneas but also the snoring as it represents airway narrowing as well.

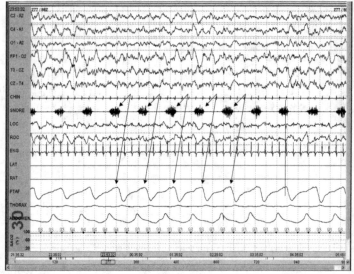

FIGURE 6.30. This is a 30-sec epoch demonstrating snoring.

S noring can occur without associated apneas. When snoring is not associated with apneas, arousals, or sleep complaints, it is referred to as primary snoring. In the sample above, notice that snoring occurs with every breath (*arrows*), but there is no associated apnea, hypopnea, desaturation, or arousal. Typically, snoring occurs at the peak of inspiration (*line*).

ABNORMALITIES OF AROUSAL

Arousal from sleep may occur for many different reasons. Polygraphic recordings demonstrate the arousal through EEG and EMG, while the underlying etiology can usually be demonstrated by monitoring oxygenation and airflow for the presence of apneas/hypopneas, snoring, or by monitors that detect leg movements or nocturnal behaviors.

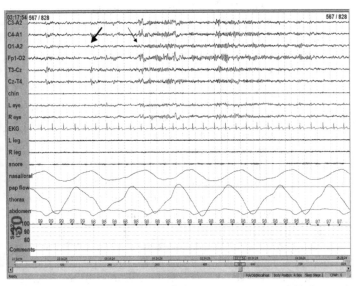

FIGURE 6.31. This is a 30-sec epoch demonstrating an unexplained arousal.

Arousals are scored based on changes in the EEG. The AASM has published rules on scoring arousals. An arousal is scored when there is an abrupt change in EEG frequency including theta, alpha, and frequencies greater than 16 Hz (but not spindles). This is subject to the following 12 rules:

1. The patient must be asleep for at least 10 sec before an arousal can be scored.
2. There must be at least 10 sec of sleep between two arousals.
3. There must be at least 3 sec of EEG frequency shift (known as the 3-sec rule).
4. An arousal from NREM sleep can occur without an increase in EMG activity.
5. An arousal from REM sleep must be accompanied by increase in EMG activity.
6. An increase in EMG by itself is not sufficient to score an arousal.
7. Delta waves, K complexes, or artifacts cannot be included in the 3 sec needed to score an arousal.
8. Pen blocking can be included in the arousal if it is contiguous to one (this applies to paper recordings).
9. Contiguous EEG and EMG changes cannot be combined in reaching the 3-sec duration criteria.
10. Alpha activity intrusion into sleep must be at least 3 sec to be scored as an arousal.
11. Sleep stage transitions cannot be scored as arousals.
12. When arousals occur in association with apneas/hypopneas, snoring, or leg movements, they are scored as associated with the same. If there is no apparent cause, they are scored as unexplained arousals. In the example shown in Figure 6.31, there is a clear change of frequency to the alpha range that lasts about 10 sec (*arrow*). Preceding the arousal are at least 10 sec of stage II sleep (*thick arrow*). Since it is not associated with either a respiratory or leg movement event, it is scored as an unexplained arousal.

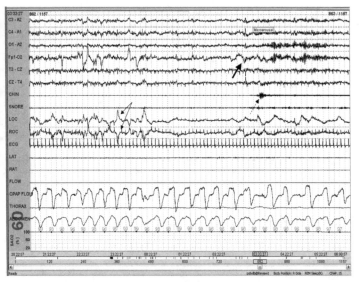

FIGURE 6.32. This is a 60-sec epoch demonstrating REM sleep, as indicated by the rapid eye movements (*thin arrows*). There is a subsequent arousal manifest as increase in the EEG frequencies (*thick arrow*) and increase of chin EMG (*dashed arrow*).

As noted previously, arousals from REM sleep must be accompanied by an increase in EMG, whereas arousals from NREM sleep do not need a concomitant increase in EMG. It must be remembered that an increase in EMG without an EEG change cannot be scored as an arousal, regardless the stage of sleep.

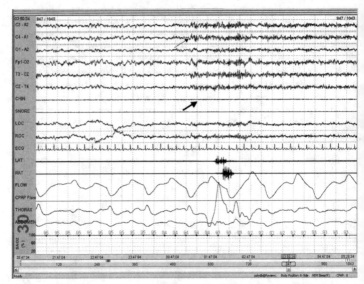

FIGURE 6.33. This is a 30-sec epoch of REM sleep demonstrating a shift in EEG frequencies that is not an arousal.

The AASM criteria specify that arousals from REM sleep must not only have a shift in EEG frequencies, but also an increase in EMG. In the figure above, there is a clear shift of EEG frequencies (*thin arrow*), but no increase in concurrent EMG (*thick arrow*). Consequently, this cannot be scored as an arousal.

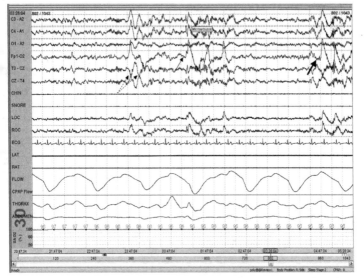

FIGURE 6.34. This is a 30-sec epoch demonstrating a single arousal from stage II sleep in the center of the page manifest as an increase in EEG frequencies (*thin arrow*). Note that the run of K complexes (*dashed arrows*) is not scored as an arousal.

Two consecutive arousals must have at least 10 sec of intervening sleep. Additionally, delta waves and K complexes cannot be including in the 3-sec duration rule. There is an additional episode of increase in EEG frequencies toward the end of the page (*thick arrow*). This also meets the 3-sec rule; however, since there is only about 8 sec of sleep intervening between the two events, the second cannot be scored as an arousal.

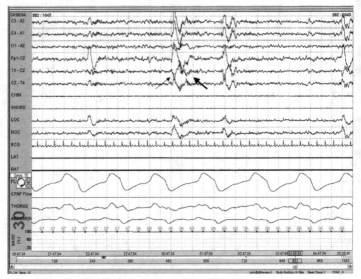

FIGURE 6.35. This is a 30-sec epoch of stage II sleep with a K complex (*thin arrow*) followed by an EEG frequency shift (*thick arrow*), which does not meet criteria for an arousal.

To be scored as an arousal, the shift in EEG frequencies must last at least 3 sec. If artifacts, delta waves, and K complexes occur before an EEG frequency shift, they are not counted toward the 3-sec rule. In the figure above, the EEG frequency shift is less than 3 sec in duration, and consequently cannot be scored as an arousal.

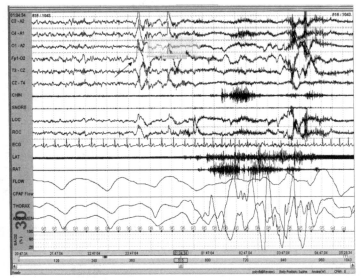

FIGURE 6.36. This is a 30-sec epoch demonstrating an awakening that occurs about the tenth second (*arrow*) that persist for >15 sec.

When the waking background returns for at least 30 sec, it is referred to as an awakening. Practically, if more than 15 sec of an epoch represent wakefulness, the whole epoch will be scored as stage W or awakening.

CHAPTER 6

PERIODIC LIMB MOVEMENTS

Movements recorded from the legs and less frequently the arms may normally be seen during sleep, although they may also occur with respiratory abnormalities. These movements may interfere with sleep and result in sleep disorders.

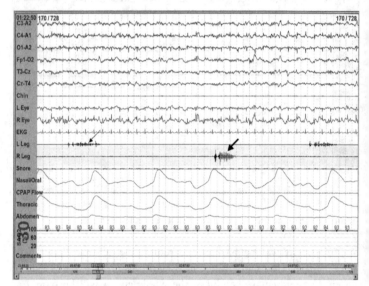

FIGURE 6.37. This is a 30-sec epoch demonstrating PLMS that occur asynchronously in the left (*thin arrow*) and right (*thick arrow*) legs. The first movement (*thin arrow*) lasts about 3 sec, and 11 sec later is followed by a second movement (*thick arrow*).

Periodic leg movements of sleep (PLMS) are recorded during sleep with two EEG cup electrodes placed 2 to 4 cm apart on the anterior tibialis muscle bilaterally. Each leg is recorded in a separate channel. Most periodic movements consist of dorsiflexion of the big toe, but occasionally this can be associated with dorsiflexion of the ankle and flexion of the knee. At times, similar movements can be noted in the arms. These movements are stereotypical and can occur for long periods of time. Asynchrony is common. To differentiate them from muscle jerks and irregular movements, the AASM has published guidelines for scoring PLMS. These guidelines state that at least five movements must occur in a series before counting can start. Each movement must last between 0.5 and 5.0 sec, and movements must be separated by 5 to 90 sec.

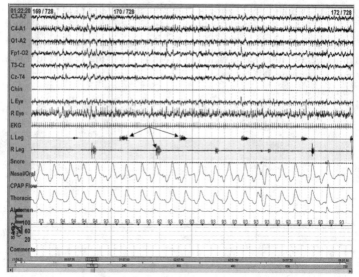

FIGURE 6.38. This is a 2-min epoch demonstrating PLMS. Note the periodicity that is evident with each movement separated by 7 to 11 sec (*arrows*).

Because of the time separating PLMS and their periodicity, they are often best seen with a longer time base (i.e., 2-min epoch). The figure above is from the same patient as the previous sample.

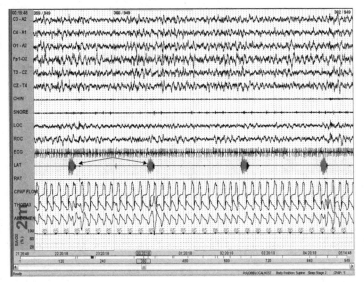

FIGURE 6.39. This is a 2-min epoch demonstrating unilateral PLMS occurring only in the left leg 25 to 30 sec apart (*arrows*).

Both legs must be monitored in a PSG with electrodes on the anterior tibialis muscles, as discussed previously. This is because occasionally leg movements will be unilateral and may not be detected if only one leg is monitored.

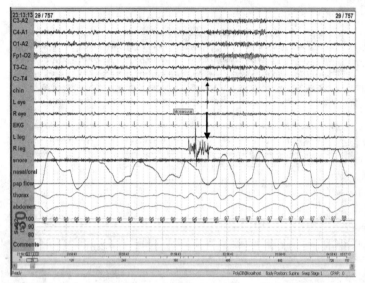

FIGURE 6.40. This is a 30-sec epoch demonstrating a leg movement associated with an arousal (*thin arrow*) that starts at the termination of the leg movement (*thick arrow*).

Leg movements may be associated with arousals or awakenings. The AASM has proposed rules for scoring leg movements associated with arousals. The arousal (a frequency shift in the EEG lasting at least 3 sec) must occur concurrently or within 1 to 2 sec after the termination of the leg movement.

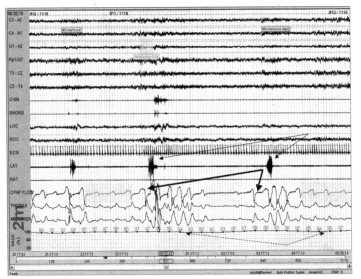

FIGURE 6.41. This is a 2-min epoch demonstrating PLMS in the left leg. The latter two leg movements (*thin arrows*) occur at the termination of a hypopnea and obstructive apnea (*thick arrows*). The respiratory events are also associated with oxygen desaturations (*dashed arrows*).

Periodic movements can be associated with apneas and hypopneas that often occur at the termination of the respiratory event. The AASM recommends that these movements be classified as movements related to respiratory events. Periodically, a respiratory event will terminate with a movement and an arousal. It becomes difficult to determine if the arousal is due to the respiratory event or leg movement, and the interpreter must rely on the clinical history in deciding the primary cause. Often when both respiratory events and PLMS are present in a single patient, the respiratory events are addressed by treatment first.

CARDIAC ARRHYTHMIAS

Arrhythmias may be encountered during sleep evaluations that reflect changes in heart rate or heart rhythm. Significant apneas or disorders of respiration may produce hypoxia that produces changes in the electrocardiogram.

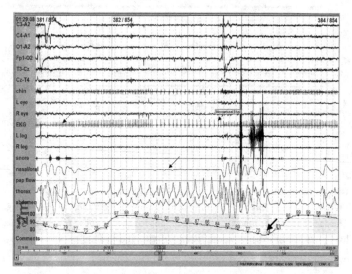

FIGURE 6.42. This is a 2-min epoch demonstrating bradyarrhythmia associated with a prolonged obstructive apnea (*thin arrow*) associated with a severe desaturation (*thick arrow*). Before the start of the apnea, the heart rate is approximately 100 beats per minute (*dashed arrow*), and this slows to about 50 beats per minute toward the end of the apnea (*dotted arrow*).

In addition to normal heart rate and rhythm changes during sleep, arrhythmias are frequently seen. They occur due to imbalances between sympathetic and parasympathetic tone. The most common of these is severe sinus bradycardia, atrioventricular block, and sinus arrest. Hypoxia produced by the apnea is thought to induce these arrhythmias. During a PSG, only one channel of ECG is recorded, and if significant abnormalities are noted, a 12-lead ECG should be ordered.

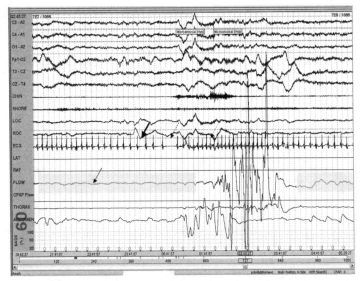

FIGURE 6.43. This is a 60-sec epoch demonstrating bradyarrhythmia and a sinus pause associated with a prolonged obstructive apnea (*thin arrow*) associated with a bradyarrhythmia (*thick arrow*). Note that the oxygen saturation channel is malfunctioning.

As noted previously, bradyarrhythmias are often seen with obstructive apneas. In severe cases, sinus pauses can occur. This is particularly likely in REM sleep due to increased parasympathetic tone, which causes further slowing of the heart rate. In this sample, the patient is in REM sleep in the first half of the epoch as manifest by the rapid eye movement. In the figure above, toward the end of the apnea, a sinus pause of almost 3 sec is noted (*dashed arrow*). At the termination of the apnea, there is a compensatory tachycardia (*dotted arrow*) and an arousal.

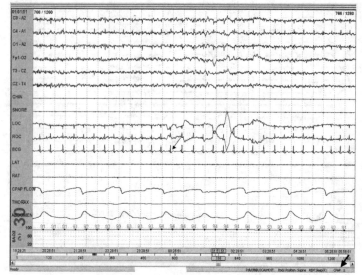

FIGURE 6.44. This is a 30-sec epoch from the same patient as the previous sample demonstrating resolution of the bradyarrhythmia and sinus pauses (*thin arrow*) with CPAP at a pressure of 11 cm H$_2$O (*thick arrow*).

The bradyarrhythmias and sinus pauses that occur with obstructive sleep apnea can often be effectively treated with CPAP. Prior to placement of a permanent cardiac pacing device for bradyarrhythmias, obstructive sleep apnea should be considered, and if present, CPAP treatment should be used. This sample is from the same patient as Figure 6.43.

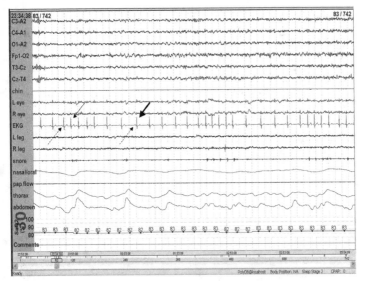

FIGURE 6.45. This is a 30-sec epoch showing sinus arrhythmia. Note that the heart rate varies between 120 (*thin arrow*) and 85 (*thick arrow*) beats per minute. The presence of P waves (*dashed arrows*) makes this a sinus arrhythmia.

Sinus arrhythmia is a frequently observed heart rhythm abnormality in sleep. It may or may not be associated with respiratory events. Sinus arrhythmia may occur in normal individuals with heart rates dropping to 40 beats per minutes. Sinus pauses of up to 2 sec have also been noted.

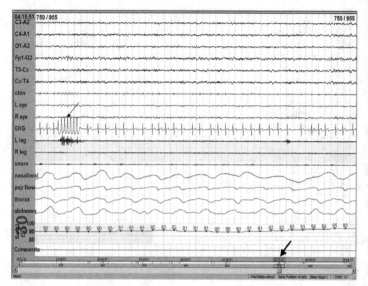

FIGURE 6.46. This is a 30-sec epoch demonstrating a run of ventricular tachycardia.

Whether ventricular arrhythmias increase or decrease in sleep is disputed. When they do occur, they are most likely in the early morning hours. These arrhythmias can occur in patients who do not have apneas and desaturations. It has been suggested that sudden death in sleep, which tends to occur more often in the early morning hours, occurs due to ventricular arrhythmias. In the figure above taken from a patient with ischemic heart disease and being evaluated for obstructive sleep apnea, a 7-beat run of ventricular tachycardia is noted (*thin arrow*). Note that this arrhythmia occurred at 4:15 AM (*thick arrow*). Significant respiratory disturbance was not noted in this study.

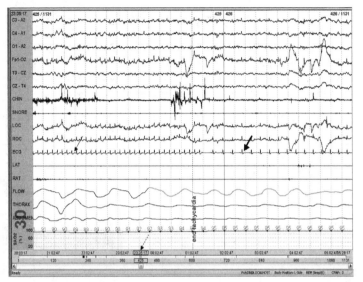

FIGURE 6.47. This is a 30-sec epoch demonstrating a run of supraventricular tachycardia with a rate of approximately 180 beats per minute (*thin arrow*) that terminates toward the middle of the epoch and replaced by normal sinus rhythm at 85 beats per minute (*thick arrow*).

Supraventricular tachycardias have a bimodal circadian peak, between 6:00 AM and 12:00 PM and between 6:00 PM and 12:00 AM. During the latter peak, changes in autonomic tone are thought to be causative. The time of the arrhythmia is noted during the recording and is seen in the above example to occur at 11:35 PM (*dashed arrow*).

EPILEPTIC DISCHARGES

Individuals with nighttime spells may have seizures as the underlying cause. Epileptiform discharges may be encountered on the EEG during PSG, although differentiating pathological spikes from artifact merits special consideration. If seizures are a strong consideration, using an expanded montage may be helpful.

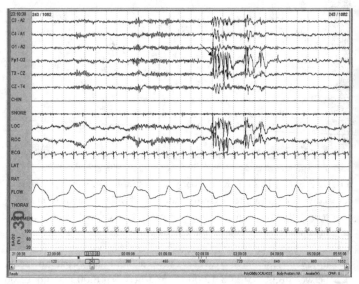

FIGURE 6.48. This is a 30-sec epoch demonstrating spikes.

Identifying spikes in a PSG viewed in 30-sec epochs is difficult because artifacts can appear as spikes. With a restricted number of EEG electrodes, localization of spikes is also very difficult. When there is a suspicion of spikes in a PSG, the relevant section should be reviewed in 10-sec epochs. If the spikes appear epileptiform in the 10-sec epochs, localization should not be attempted due to the small number of EEG channels. Rather a standard EEG should be ordered. If there is a high suspicion of epilepsy in a patient undergoing a PSG, consideration should be given to applying a full set of EEG electrodes and acquiring an 18-channel EEG during the PSG. In the patient shown above, there was no history of epilepsy and these sharp discharges (*arrow*) were seen on multiple occasions. Because of their morphology, they raised the suspicion of epileptiform discharges and were viewed in a10-sec epoch (see next sample).

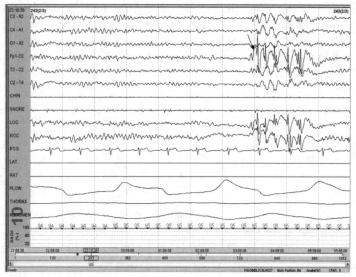

FIGURE 6.49. This is a 10-sec epoch demonstrating spikes.

Here the spikes noted in the previous sample are viewed in a 10-sec epoch. Although the morphology can now be better described as a spike and wave discharge (*arrow*), no comment can be made about localization. The amplitude appears to be the highest in the Fp1-O2 derivation; however, this is because that derivation has the longest interelectrode distance. The spike and wave discharge is also seen in the EOG. Since it is in phase, it is not caused by an eye movement. This patient underwent a 21 channel sleep-deprived EEG a few days after the PSG and was noted to have generalized polyspike and wave discharges.

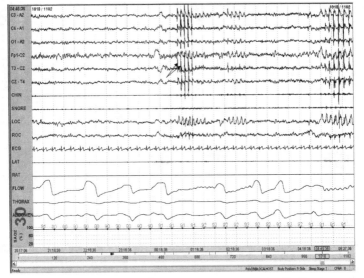

FIGURE 6.50. This is a 30-sec epoch demonstrating runs of spikes.

Spikes can be difficult to differentiate from artifacts on a PSG due to the 30-sec time window and restricted EEG montage. Steps outlined previously can help differentiate epileptiform discharges from other findings. In the figure above, bursts of 3- and 4-Hz discharges (*arrows*) were noted frequently during the PSG, particularly in light stages of sleep.

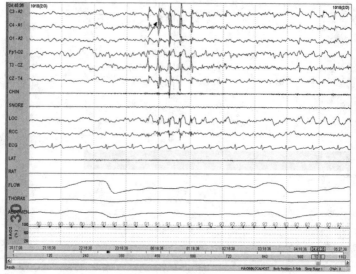

FIGURE 6.51. This is a 10-sec epoch demonstrating epileptiform discharges.

Changing the paper speed to 10 sec per epoch helps evaluate the morphology of the spike discharge. This sample represents the middle 10 sec of the previous sample. The discharges have polyspike morphology (*arrow*) and clearly look epileptiform. However, an epileptiform appearing PSG should be followed by an EEG to confirm that the patient has epileptiform discharges.

MISCELLANEOUS FINDINGS

Many other patterns can be seen on PSG. Some have diagnostic significance, while others do not. The presence of some findings may support additional testing.

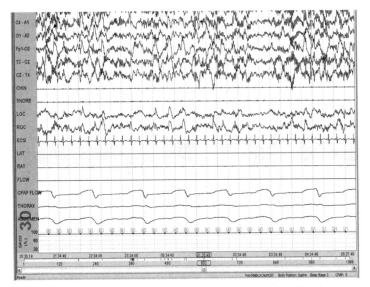

FIGURE 6.52. This is a 30-sec epoch demonstrating alpha-delta sleep pattern. The alpha activity can be seen overriding the delta waves (*arrow*).

In the alpha-delta sleep pattern there is persistence of alpha frequency activity in NREM sleep. The distribution of the alpha activity is more pervasive than normal alpha rhythm, and the frequency is usually slower. Underlying sleep spindles, K complexes, and delta waves confirm the true stage of sleep. Earlier studies noted the occurrence of this pattern in patients with chronic pain syndromes, fibromyalgia, and nonrestorative sleep. However, more recently, this association and the significance of alpha delta sleep have been questioned. In the author's practice, when this pattern is seen, it is described, but no clinical significance is attributed.

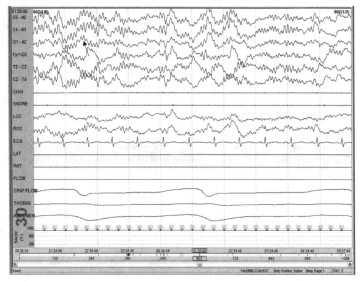

FIGURE 6.53. This is a 10-sec epoch of alpha-delta sleep; it is the first 10 sec of the previous sample.

This sample is displayed at a paper speed of 30 mm/sec. It clearly shows 10-Hz activity superimposed on slower delta frequencies (*arrow*). When alpha frequencies are seen in non-REM sleep, it is often useful to change the paper speed to 30 mm/sec to better visualize the various frequencies present and determine the correct stage of sleep. Based on the underlying delta activity, this epoch was scored as stage III.

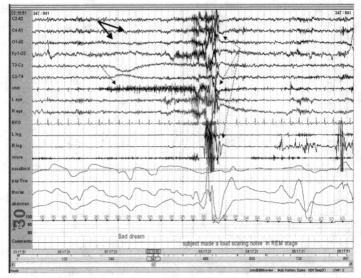

FIGURE 6.54. This is a 30-sec epoch demonstrating increased EMG activity during REM sleep creating excessive EMG tonic activity (*thin arrow*) in the chin channel during REM sleep. REM sleep is manifest during this epoch by a low-amplitude, mixed-frequency EEG activity (*thick arrow*).

In REM sleep, there is muscle atonia. This is manifest on PSG with the chin EMG activity at its lowest level of any stage of sleep. REM sleep behavior disorder (RBD) is a REM sleep parasomnia that occurs due to loss of the normal muscle atonia in REM sleep. This is manifest by an increase in phasic and tonic EMG activity during REM sleep. Soon after the EMG activity starts, the patient has a spell of yelling and movement (as noted by the technologist). This is manifest by EMG artifact (*dashed arrows*) in the above example. Immediately after the episode, the patient returns to sleep.

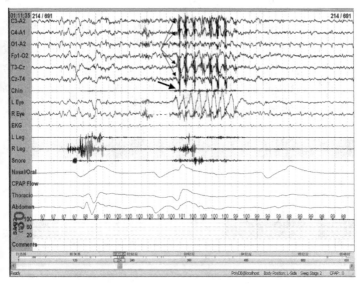

FIGURE 6.55. This is a 30-sec epoch demonstrating bruxism.

Bruxism can occur in both NREM and REM sleep. It manifests on PSG as bursts of EMG activity best seen in the temporal or ear leads due to their proximity to the jaw. By virtue of their location under the mandible, the chin EMG electrodes do not record the bursts of activity as well as the temporal electrodes. The EMG activity associated with bruxism occurs at a rate of 1 Hz and each burst lasts at least 5 sec. Chewing artifact can appear similar; however, it is not seen in sleep and usually lasts longer than bruxism. In the example above, the burst of EMG activity is noted best in the temporal and ear electrodes (*thin arrows*). Note that the patient is in stage II sleep, and the burst of EMG activity occurs at a rate of approximately 1 Hz, making it consistent with bruxism. Minimal activity is not noted in the chin EMG lead (*thick arrow*).

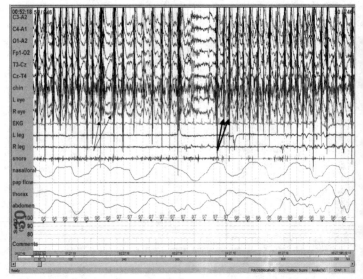

FIGURE 6.56. This is a 30-sec epoch demonstrating chewing artifact. Note that the frequency of the artifact varies from 1 per second (*thin arrows*) to about 2 per second (*thick arrows*).

Chewing results in EMG artifact in EEG electrodes. Like bruxism, this activity is best noted in temporal and ear electrodes because of their proximity to the mandible. However, at times, all electrodes may be involved. The patient is awake during chewing; however, due to the pervasive nature of the artifact, recognizing the underlying EEG may be difficult. The frequency of the artifact is more variable than bruxism. In this sample, a high-amplitude EMG artifact is seen in all EEG channels, as well as in chin EMG and EOG channels. Although difficult to tell from the EEG, the patient is awake (as noted on video).

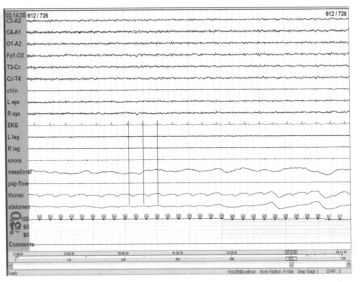

FIGURE 6.57. This is a 30-sec epoch demonstrating a ballistocardiographic artifact that is noted in the thoracic channel. The nature of this artifact can be confirmed by noting its synchrony with the ECG (*lines*).

Ballistocardiographic artifacts occur when there is movement of electrodes induced by cardiac or vascular pulsations. Consequently, this artifact is always harmonious with the cardiac rhythm. Ballistocardiographic artifact can be seen in any channel and is particularly common in EEG leads. This is particularly likely if the electrode has been placed on or near a blood vessel. Thoracic and abdominal belts used to monitor respiratory effort can also show ballistocardiographic artifact from pulsations of the heart and aorta. This artifact should not be confused with the presence of respiratory effort as the deflections occur at a faster rate than those associated with respirations.

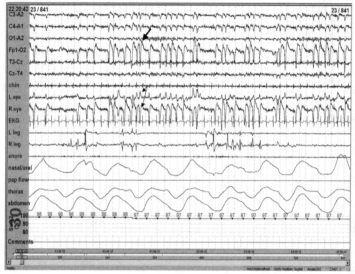

FIGURE 6.58. This is a 30-sec epoch demonstrating frequent eye blinks.

The eye acts as an electrically charged dipole with the cornea being positive relative to the electronegativity of the retina. Whenever the eye moves, the electrical charge is recorded by not only the EOG but also nearby EEG leads (i.e., Fp1). In the example above, wakefulness is noted with frequent eye blinks. They produce an out of phase deflection in the eye leads (*thin arrows*). A high-amplitude discharge is noted in the Fp1-O2 channel as well (*thick arrow*). This deflection does not suggest that the discharge is produced by the brain and instead, the proximity of the Fp1 electrode to the eye is what results in the deflection.

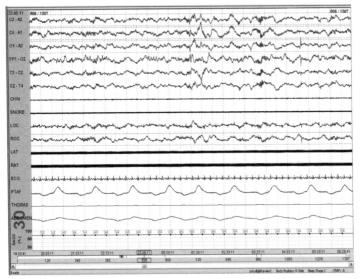

FIGURE 6.59. This is a 30-sec epoch demonstrating an electrical artifact in both leg leads.

If electrodes are not applied securely, they can be dislodged during the study. This produces an impedance mismatch between two electrodes and compromises the common mode rejection ratio of the differential amplifier. The result of this is presence of 60-Hz or other electrical noise in the channel. In this sample, frequent leg movements resulted in slight dislodgement of one electrode on each leg. The impaired electrode contact with skin resulted in an impedance mismatch and a 60-Hz artifact in the leg leads. Subsequent leg movements could not be reliably recorded because of the artifact.

MULTIPLE SLEEP LATENCY TEST

The multiple sleep latency test (MSLT) is a daytime sleep study in which an individual undergoes repeat naps serially at scheduled time intervals during the day to evaluate complaints of excessive daytime sleepiness. This test is an adjunct to overnight polysomnography to arrive at the specific diagnosis necessary for proper treatment.

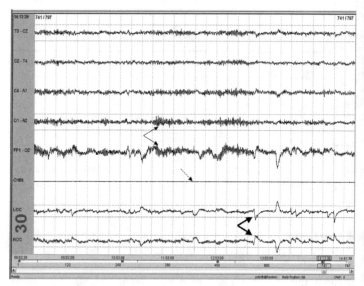

FIGURE 6.60. This 30-sec epoch from a multiple sleep latency test (MSLT) demonstrates wakefulness with alpha activity in the occipital channels (*thin arrows*) and rapid eye movements (*thick arrows*). The chin EMG (*dashed arrow*) is of higher amplitude than when the patient falls asleep.

The multiple sleep latency test (MSLT) is a daytime sleep study composed of several naps obtained several times during the day. The first nap starts 2 hr after awakening from nocturnal sleep. The patient is asked to sleep. If sleep does not occur, the test is ended in 20 min; if it does, the patient is allowed to sleep for 15 min. This procedure is repeated at 2-hr intervals four to five times throughout the day.

Sleep onset is scored at the first 30-sec epoch of any stage of sleep. For each nap, sleep-onset latency and whether the patient had REM sleep is noted. The mean sleep latency of all the naps is calculated and the number of naps with REM sleep, known as sleep-onset REM periods (SOREMP), is noted. The montage for an MSLT is different than that used for a PSG. Typically only EEG, chin EMG, and EOG channels are used without respiratory monitors and leg EMG.

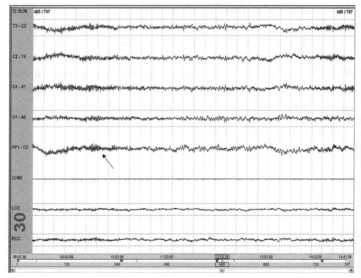

FIGURE 6.61. This is a 30-sec epoch of an MSLT showing sleep onset.

As noted before, sleep onset in an MSLT is scored at the first epoch of any stage of sleep. This is usually stage I and is manifest with loss of the alpha rhythm and slow eye movements. A mean sleep latency of less than 5 min (some investigators use 8 min) is suggestive of pathological hypersomnolence, whereas greater than 10 min is normal, and between 5 and 10 min, is considered indeterminate. In the figure above, there is loss of the alpha activity in the seventh second (*arrow*). Since more than 15 sec of this page has stage I sleep, this epoch is scored as sleep onset. Sleep latency is calculated by calculating the difference between lights off and sleep onset times.

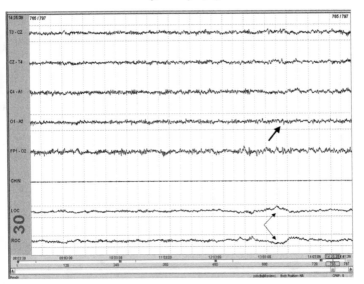

FIGURE 6.62. This is a 30-sec epoch of an MSLT showing stage I sleep with slow, rolling eye movements (*thin arrows*) and mixed-frequency EEG activity (*thick arrow*).

Features of stage I sleep in a MSLT are the same as in PSG. In addition to the loss of alpha rhythm, there is appearance of slow, rolling eye movements, mixed-frequency activity in the 2- to 7-Hz range, and finally vertex waves.

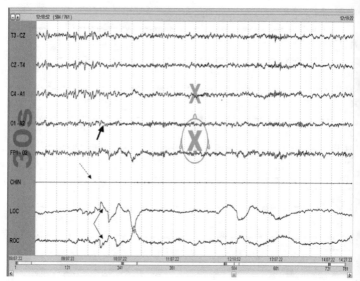

FIGURE 6.63. This is a 30-sec epoch of an MSLT showing a SOREMP.

In addition to noting the sleep-onset latency, whether or not REM sleep occurs must also be noted for each MSLT nap. The number of naps with SOREMP should be noted. If two or more naps have SOREMP, the study is considered suggestive of narcolepsy. The mean sleep latency is less than 5 min in narcolepsy. In the figure above, rapid eye movements start in the seventh second (*thin arrows*). Simultaneously, the EEG changes to mixed-frequency activity (*thick arrow*) noted in REM sleep. The chin EMG is lower than the remainder of the record (*dashed arrow*) This nap is scored as a SOREMP.

ADDITIONAL RESOURCES

AASM. Sleep-related breathing disorders in adults: recommendations for syndrome definition and measurement techniques in clinical research. The Report of an American Academy of Sleep Medicine Task Force. *Sleep* 199;22(5):667–689.

Arand D, Bonnet M, Hurwitz T, et al. The clinical use of the MSLT and MWT. *Sleep* 22005;8(1):123–144.

ASDA. EEG arousals: scoring rules and examples: a preliminary report from the Sleep Disorders Atlas Task Force of the American Sleep Disorders Association. *Sleep* 1992;15(2): 173–184.

ASDA. Recording and scoring leg movements. The Atlas Task Force. *Sleep* 1993;16(8):748–759.

Berry RB, Geyer JD, Carney PR. Introduction to sleep and sleep monitoring—the basics. In: Carney PR, Berry RB, Geyer JD, eds. *Clinical Sleep Disorders*. Lippincott Williams & Wilkins, Philadelphia, 2005:3–26.

Carskadon MA, Dement WC, Mitler MM, et al. Guidelines for the multiple sleep latency test (MSLT): a standard measure of sleepiness. *Sleep* 1986;9(4):519–524.

Gillis AM, Flemons WW. Cardiac arrhythmias during sleep. In: Kryger MH, Roth T, Dement WC, eds. *Principles and Practice of Sleep Medicine*. 2nd ed. Saunders, London, 1994;847–860.

Littner MR, Kushida C, Wise M, et al. Practice parameters for clinical use of the multiple sleep latency test and the maintenance of wakefulness test. *Sleep* 2005;28(1):113–121.

Mitler MM, Poceta S, Bigby BG. Sleep scoring technique. In: Chokroverty S, ed. *Sleep Disorders Medicine: Basic Science, Technical Considerations, and Clinical Aspects*. 2nd ed. Butterworth Heinemann, Boston, 1999:245–262.

Parisi RA. Respiration and respiratory function: Technique of recording and evaluation. In: Chokroverty S, ed. *Sleep Disorders Medicine: Basic Science, Technical Considerations, and Clinical Aspects*. 2nd ed. Butterworth Heinemann, Boston, 1999:215–221.

Radtke RA. Sleep disorders: laboratory evaluation. In: Ebersole JS, Pedley TA, eds. *Current Practice of Clinical Electroencephalography*. 3rd ed. Lippincott Williams & Wilkins, Philadelphia, 2003:803–832.

Rechtschaffen A, Kales A, eds. A manual of standardized terminology, techniques and scoring system for sleep stages of human subjects. Los Angeles, UCLA Brain Information Service/Brain Research Institute, 1968.

Shamsuzzaman AS, Gersh BJ, Somers VK. Obstructive sleep apnea: implications for cardiac and vascular disease. *JAMA* 2003;290(14):1906–1914.

Shepard JWJ. (1991). *Atlas of Sleep Medicine*. Futura, Mount Kisco, NY, 1991.

Wittig RM, Zorick FJ, Blumer D. Disturbed sleep in patients complaining of chronic pain. *J Nerv Ment Dis* 1982;170(7):429–431.

Neurophysiologic Intraoperative Monitoring

AATIF M. HUSAIN

Neurophysiologic intraoperative monitoring (NIOM) is increasingly being used to reduce neurologic morbidity associated with surgeries that are performed where the nervous system is at risk. NIOM allows assessment of neurologic function when the patient cannot be examined. Often the neurophysiologist is able to alert the surgeon of impending injury and potential neurologic sequelae, allowing the surgeon to modify or reverse the procedure. Several techniques can be used to monitor the integrity of the nervous system during surgery, and these are chosen depending on the part of the nervous system that is at risk and type of surgery. Common modalities utilized during NIOM include brainstem auditory evoked potentials (BAEP), somatosensory evoked potentials (SEP), transcranial electrical motor evoked potentials (MEP), electromyography (EMG), and electroencephalography (EEG). Often more than one modality is used; this is known as multimodality monitoring. In this chapter, each modality is shown separately for illustration purposes, although in clinical practice many different types of monitoring techniques are used simultaneously.

BRAINSTEM AUDITORY EVOKED POTENTIALS

Brainstem auditory evoked potential (BAEP) monitoring is used whenever there is potential for injury to the vestibulocochlear nerve or its pathways. Microvascular decompression (MVD) for trigeminal neuralgia, hemifacial spasms, and cerebellopontine angle (CPA) tumor surgery often utilize BAEP monitoring intraoperatively, although it may also be used during other types of brainstem surgery. BAEP monitoring ipsilateral to the side of surgery has been shown to reduce the incidence of hearing loss associated with MVD surgeries. Changes in the latencies and amplitudes of the wave I and wave V from baseline are observed. The contralateral median nerve somatosensory evoked potential (SEP) is also periodically monitored to evaluate conduction in the dorsal column pathways in the brainstem that lie close to the vestibulocochlear pathway. Multimodality monitoring is particularly useful in CPA tumor surgery, and periodically, the contralateral BAEP and ipsilateral median SEP are also checked for comparison purposes.

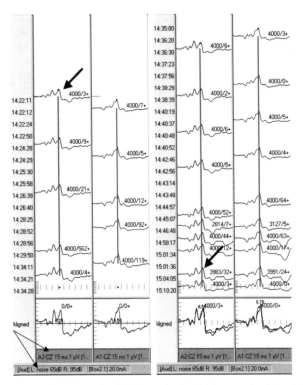

FIGURE 7.1. Intraoperative BAEP monitoring (right ear stimulation) showing no significant change in the latency and amplitude of wave V (*thick arrow*) during microvascular decompression (MVD) surgery for right trigeminal neuralgia. Note the stimulation parameters at the bottom of the graph (*thin arrows*). The vertical line is drawn on the wave V. Notice the consistency with which the wave V falls on this line, indicating no significant change in latency.

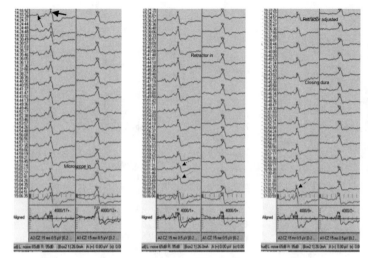

FIGURE 7.2. Intraoperative BAEP monitoring data in a patient undergoing MVD for right trigeminal neuralgia that shows an increase in wave V latency and a 50% decrease in amplitude.

During BAEP monitoring a wave V latency prolongation of 1 msec or an amplitude decrement of 50% is considered significant. The latency shift is considered more important. Three possible mechanisms can cause a change in the BAEP; first are technical issues, then global physiological changes (anesthesia or blood pressure fluctuation), and finally surgically induced change. During MVD surgery the cerebellum is retracted to expose the CPA, which may cause a stretch injury to the vestibulocochlear nerve and hearing loss if severe. In the figure above, waves I (*thin arrow*) and V (*thick arrow*) are initially identified. Soon after placement of the cerebellar retractor, there is prolongation of the wave V latency (notice the dot placed on the peak of wave V at baseline). The maximum latency prolongation is 0.6 msec, which does not reach the critical 1-msec point at which the surgeon must be alerted (*dashed arrows*), however, there is a significant decrease in the amplitude (>50%) (*dotted arrow*). The surgeon is alerted, and he repositions the cerebellar retractor. When the retractor is removed, the wave V gradually returns to baseline (*dash and dot arrow*). The return of the BAEP to near baseline suggests that permanent damage to the vestibulocochlear pathway ipsilateral to the side of surgery did not occur.

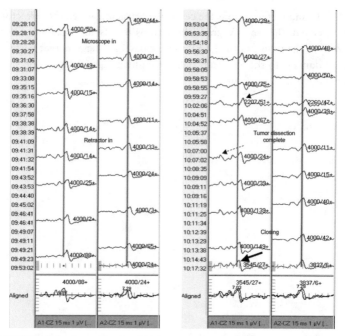

FIGURE 7.3. Intraoperative BAEP monitoring data in a patient undergoing resection of a left acoustic neuroma showing a wave V latency prolongation of 1.5 msec and amplitude reduction of more than 50%.

A 1-msec prolongation of wave V latency is considered significant, and the surgeon should be alerted. A persistent 1 msec or worsening latency shift is more likely to be associated with postoperative hearing loss. More recent data suggest that even smaller latency shifts may be clinically significant in patients with CPA tumors. In the figure above, notice that the vertical line is over the wave V at baseline; at the time of tumor dissection, there is maximal shift of the wave V (*thin arrow*). By the end of the surgery, the latency of wave V is close to baseline signified by the vertical line (*thick arrow*). Presence of wave I at the time of maximal wave V shift verifies the adequacy of stimulation (*dashed arrow*).

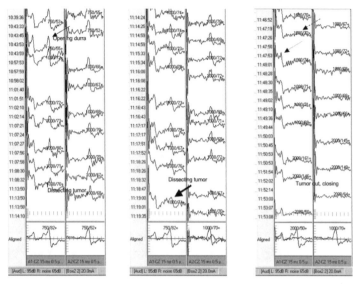

FIGURE 7.4. Intraoperative BAEP monitoring showing loss of wave V during left CPA tumor dissection without return by the end of the surgery.

The loss of the wave V waveform is most severe type of change that can occur with intraoperative BAEP monitoring. If it does not return by the end of the surgery, the patient is likely to have postoperative hearing loss. However, the loss of the wave V is not incompatible with preserved hearing (false-positive). When complete loss of wave V occurs suddenly, it is usually due to interruption of the vascular supply of the vestibulocochlear nerve. If the loss is gradual, the etiology is more likely to be either mechanical or thermal trauma to the nerve. In the figure above, there is a robust wave V at the start of the case (*thin arrow*); however, as dissection proceeds there is gradual loss of amplitude (*thick arrow*) and eventually complete loss of wave V (*dashed arrow*) that does not return by the end of the surgery. The preserved wave I (*dotted arrow*) confirms that this change is not due to technical reasons.

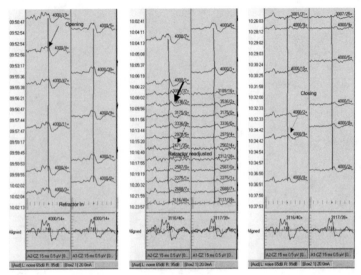

FIGURE 7.5. Intraoperative BAEP monitoring during MVD for right trigeminal neuralgia showing loss of wave V with return by the end of the surgery.

Transient loss of wave V followed by recovery before the end of the surgery suggests that hearing will be preserved. This is especially true in patients undergoing MVD surgery. In the figure above, wave V is noted at baseline (*thin arrow*); however, with cerebellar retraction there is gradual latency prolongation up to 0.7 msec with amplitude reduction (*thick arrow*) and eventual disappearance (*dashed arrow*). When the surgeon is notified and the retractor is removed, there is a gradual return of wave V (*dotted arrow*).

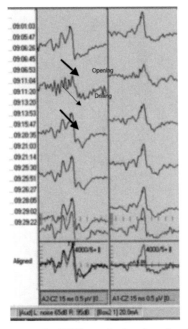

FIGURE 7.6. Intraoperative BAEP monitoring data showing loss of wave V during the noise associated with the use of a bone drill.

In addition to surgically induced changes, BAEP changes can occur due to technical issues and physiological changes. One such technical issue arises with bone drilling during exposure. The drill makes a loud noise that can mask the acoustic stimulus of the BAEP. This may cause loss of the BAEP waveforms. It is recommended that BAEP averaging be suspended during drilling. In the example above, BAEP averaging is continued during drilling. Note the lower amplitude wave V waveform (*thin arrow*). Before and after drilling, the wave V waveform is robust.

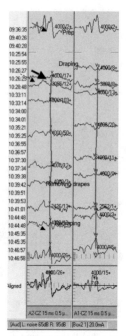

FIGURE 7.7. Intraoperative BAEP monitoring showing loss of wave V soon after draping the patient undergoing MVD for right trigeminal neuralgia.

Many technical problems can lead to loss of BAEP waveforms such as inadequacy of stimulation. A relatively common cause is kinking or clamping of the tubing used to transmit the acoustic stimulus from the sound generator to the ear. Obstruction of this tubing prevents the clicks from reaching the auditory system, and consequently a BAEP is not produced. After positioning the patient in the example above, the baseline response was obtained and revealed a robust wave V waveform (*thin arrow*). Soon after draping the patient, however, there was a sudden loss of the wave V (*thick arrow*) as well as wave I (*dashed arrows*). The absence of all BAEP waveforms suggested inadequacy of stimulation. After the clamps of the drape were removed, the BAEP response returned (*dotted arrow*).

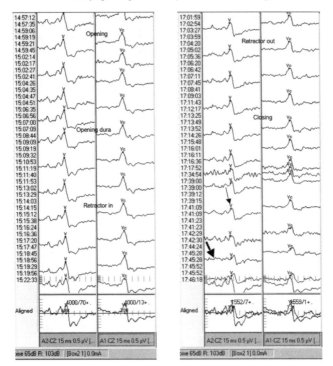

FIGURE 7.8. Intraoperative BAEP monitoring showing latency prolongation and amplitude decrement of the wave V toward the end of the surgery due to technical problems of stimulating electrode dislodgement from the ear.

The auditory stimulator can be inadvertently dislodged during surgery. This is more likely to occur when the surgery is prolonged. When the stimulating electrode is dislodged, there is a lower stimulus intensity delivered to the ear to produce the BAEP. Consequently, the BAEP may demonstrate an artifactual prolongation of the latency and reduction of the amplitude as the electrode becomes further removed from the canal. In the example above, there is gradual prolongation of latency and a drop in amplitude of the wave V waveform toward the end of the surgery (*thin arrow*). At the end of the surgery, the technologist confirmed that the stimulator tubing had been dislodged. Note that as the wave V disappears, so does the wave I, indicating a peripheral etiology for the change (*thick arrow*).

SOMATOSENSORY EVOKED POTENTIALS

Somatosensory evoked potential (SEP) monitoring is utilized for demonstrating the integrity of the large-fiber sensory tracts. During surgery, upper and lower SEPs may be used to detect changes in dorsal column function of the posterior spinal cord. Anesthesia, blood flow, and technical constraints may directly impact and produce changes in amplitude and/or latency of SEPs.

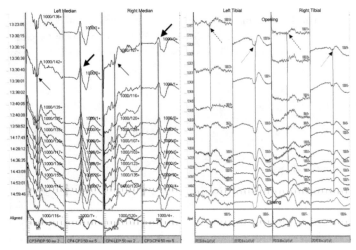

FIGURE 7.9. Intraoperative median and tibial SEP monitoring data that shows no significant change during posterior spinal fusion for scoliosis. Median nerve SEPs are used as a control.

Somatosensory evoked potential monitoring is most often used for monitoring spinal cord function, however it can also be used during surgeries on the brainstem and thoracic aorta. In scoliosis surgery, SEP monitoring has been shown to result in reduced neurological morbidity. SEPs obtained through posterior tibial nerve stimulation are used when surgery involves risk to the spinal cord below the lower cervical level. In such cases, median nerve SEPs can be used as a control. For surgeries involving risk to the upper to mid-cervical spinal cord, median or ulnar SEP is used (ulnar preferentially used if C6 to C7 region is at risk). Subcortical (P14/N18 for upper, P31/N34 for lower) and cortical (N20 for upper, P37 for lower) waveforms are followed during surgery. SEPs monitor the posterior aspect of spinal cord (dorsal columns) and therefore, are often done in conjunction with additional types of monitoring (i.e., motor evoked potentials). In Figure 7.9, both subcortical median and posterior tibial SEPs (P14, *thin arrows*; P31, *dashed arrows*) seen in the first and third columns and cortical (N20, *thick arrows*; P37, *dotted arrows*) noted in the second and fourth columns are displayed. When no significant changes in the responses are noted, neurological morbidity is not anticipated.

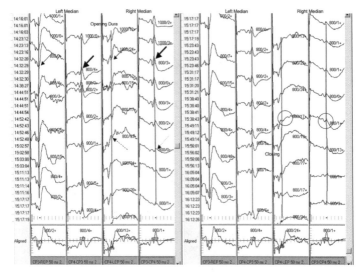

FIGURE 7.10. Intraoperative median SEP monitoring showing gradual loss of the subcortical and cortical waveforms after right sided stimulation in a patient undergoing decompression of syringomyelia.

A significant change in SEP is a 50% decrease in amplitude or a 10% increase in latency. Unlike BAEPs, with SEPs an amplitude change is more significant. When such a change occurs, and technical and general physiological causes have been excluded, the surgeon should be alerted. In the figure above, note the median SEP subcortical responses (first and third columns) and cortical responses (second and fourth columns) are displayed. At the start of the case, robust subcortical (*thin arrows*) and cortical (*thick arrows*) responses are seen. As surgery continues, there is a gradual loss of amplitude of the subcortical (*dashed arrow*) and cortical (*dotted arrow*) waveforms obtained after right-sided stimulation. At the end of surgery, these responses are almost completely lost (*circles*). The patient is likely to have postoperative dysfunction that involves the sensory pathways mediated by the dorsal columns of the right median nerve.

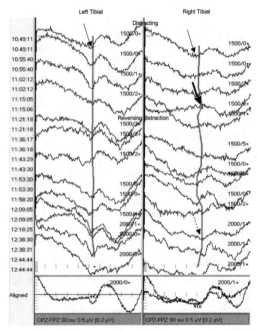

FIGURE 7.11. Intraoperative posterior tibial SEP monitoring data showing transient loss of the cortical waveform after right tibial nerve stimulation in a patient undergoing a posterior spinal fusion for scoliosis.

During scoliosis surgery implantation of hardware (sublaminar wires and hooks) and distraction can lead to spinal cord injury. Monitoring SEP allows determination of when such compromise is imminent. In the figure above, cortical (P37) waveforms (*thin arrows*) are seen at the start of distraction from right tibial nerve stimulation. However, shortly thereafter, the cortical response has a decrease in amplitude and becomes difficult to identify (*thick arrow*), and the surgeon is alerted. After the surgeon reverses the distraction, the responses improve (*dashed arrow*). Without SEP monitoring the surgeon would not have been aware of the spinal cord compromise, possibly leading to neurological morbidity.

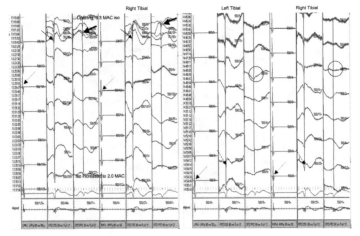

FIGURE 7.12. Intraoperative tibial SEP monitoring showing gradual loss of the cortical waveforms with use of halogenated anesthetics in a patient undergoing surgery for scoliosis.

There are many systemic factors that can affect SEP. One of the most common is anesthetics. Cortical waveforms, particularly the tibial SEP, are very sensitive to inhalation (halogenated agents and nitrous oxide) anesthetics. Concentrations of 1 minimum alveolar concentration (MAC), or above can eliminate the cortical responses. Subcortical responses are more resilient to anesthetics and often can be followed in cases in which such anesthetics are required. In the example above, when isoflurane 0.3 MAC is initially used, well-defined subcortical (*thin arrows*) and cortical (*thick arrows*) responses are seen. However, when the isoflurane is increased to 2 MAC, there is obliteration of the cortical response bilaterally (*circles*). Notice that the subcortical responses persist despite the increase in anesthetics (*dashed arrows*). The first and fourth columns are the popliteal fossa (PF) responses (*dotted arrow*), which indicates adequacy of stimulation.

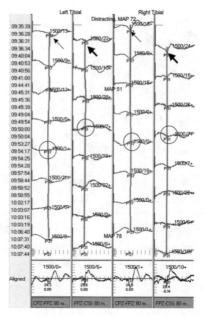

FIGURE 7.13. Intraoperative tibial SEP monitoring showing intermittent loss of cortical and subcortical waveforms with fluctuating blood pressure in a patient undergoing posterior spinal fusion for scoliosis.

A reduction in blood pressure can affect the SEP waveforms, causing a decrease in amplitude of the cortical and subcortical potentials. This is likely due to hypoperfusion of the spinal cord. In the figure above, the first and third columns display the cortical (P37) waveforms, while the second and fourth columns display the subcortical (P31/N34) waveforms. When the mean arterial pressure (MAP) is about 70 mm Hg, both cortical (*thin arrows*) and subcortical (*thick arrows*) waveforms are seen. However, when the pressure drops to about 50 mm Hg, there is significant amplitude reduction of the waveforms (*circles*). When the pressure is raised, the responses return (*dashed arrows*). In this patient, monitoring directs the anesthesiologist to maintain a relatively higher MAP.

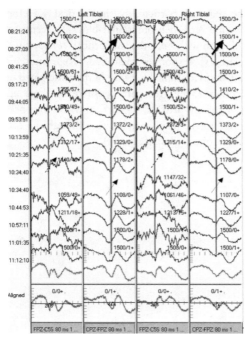

FIGURE 7.14. Intraoperative tibial SEP monitoring showing poor reproducibility of the subcortical waveforms and preserved cortical waveforms with wearing off of neuromuscular blocking agents in a patient undergoing anterior cervical decompression and fixation for spinal stenosis.

Subcortical SEPs are smaller potentials than cortical responses and are harder to resolve with averaging. With EMG contamination, subcortical waveforms are even more difficult to obtain. Consequently, if patients are not given neuromuscular-blocking agents or higher doses of anesthetic gases during surgery, often the subcortical waveforms cannot be clearly seen. With neuromuscular-blocking agents, even though SEP subcortical waveforms can be easily resolved, MEP cannot be used. On the other hand, with higher doses of anesthetic gases, although there is less EMG, the SEP waveforms' amplitude may be reduced, particularly the cortical waveforms. In the example in Figure 7.14, neuromuscular-blocking agents were initially used for intubation with both the subcortical (*thin arrows*) and cortical (*thick arrows*) responses identified. Neuromuscular-blocking agents were then discontinued because of the anticipated use of motor evoked potentials (MEP) that are sensitive to these agents. With return of the myogenic artifact, subcortical waveforms became harder to resolve and "noisy" (*dashed arrows*), although the cortical waveforms remained robust (*dotted arrows*).

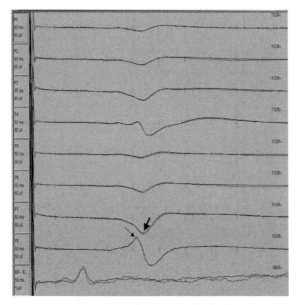

FIGURE 7.15. Intraoperative median SEP used to localize the central sulcus in a patient with left facial pain undergoing stimulator placement.

SEP has been used diagnostically to localize the central sulcus in patients undergoing neurosurgery near the motor strip. It has also been used for patients undergoing therapeutic stimulator implantations for facial pain. Recording from at least eight contacts is optimal from the exposed cortex. Contralateral median nerve SEPs are obtained sequentially from the various contacts on a grid or a strip placed across a sulcus. An N20 waveform is seen over the somatosensory cortex, while a P22 (sometimes called the P20) waveform is seen over the motor cortex. The N20 and P22 produce a "phase reversal." The central sulcus is thought to reside between the electrodes generating the highest amplitude N20/P22 complex. In the figure above, there are robust N20 (*thin arrow*) and P22 (*thick arrow*) waveforms that phase reverse at contacts 7 and 8. The central sulcus located beneath and between these contacts.

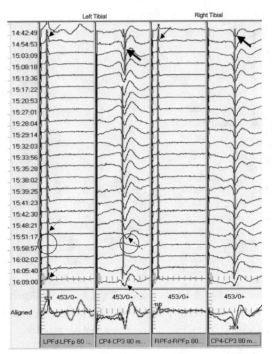

FIGURE 7.16. Intraoperative tibial SEP monitoring showing the loss of both PF (first and third column) and P37 (second and fourth column) waveforms after left-sided stimulation in a patient undergoing a thoracic laminectomy for excision of an extradural spinal lesion.

Technical issues must also be considered whenever there is a change in waveforms. Whereas physiological changes, such as anesthetic and blood pressure changes, are more likely to affect all SEP responses, technical issues are more likely to produce more restricted waveform changes. In the example above, robust PF (*thin arrows*) and P37 (*thick arrows*) responses are initially seen bilaterally. At 15:51:17 mild latency prolongation of the P37 after left tibial nerve stimulation is noted (*dashed arrow*) with an ipsilateral PF amplitude reduction (*dotted arrow*) progressing to complete absence of both the

PF and P37 responses (*circles*). Loss of the PF response suggests a technical problem with stimulation on the left side. The technologist checked the stimulating needles and found that they had been dis-lodged. Readjusting the stimulating needles resulted in return of both the PF and P37 responses (*dashed-dotted arrows*)

MOTOR EVOKED POTENTIALS

Motor evoked potentials are utilized to demonstrate integrity of the motor tracts. In this way, the corticospinal tracts are able to be monitored to help predict the likelihood of postoperative weakness. In conjunction with SEPs, the anterior and posterior portions of the spinal cord can be monitored together. Similar to SEPs, MEPs are sensitive to anesthetics and, especially, neuromuscular blockade.

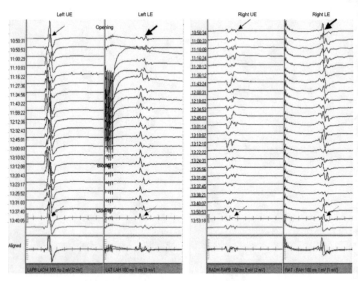

FIGURE 7.17. Intraoperative MEP monitoring showing stable responses in the upper and lower extremities during a biopsy of a cervical lesion.

Motor evoked potentials (MEPs) are obtained by electrically stimulating the brain and recording the response over the spinal cord (Direct = D and Indirect = I waves), peripheral nerves (nerve action potentials), or muscles (compound muscle action potentials, CMAP). In this way, the motor (corticospinal) tracts located in the anterior spinal cord are evaluated, and this provides a much better predictor of postoperative weakness than the SEP. Usually, recordings are made from small hand and foot muscles. Spinal recordings (for D and I waves) are seldom used owing to the invasive methods required for recording. When recording MEPs from muscles, a train of high voltage (200 to 600 V) stimuli is applied to the scalp to peripherally produce a CMAP. Large series have demonstrated the safe use of MEPs, and they are a useful adjunct to SEP monitoring. Using both modalities, both the anterior and posterior aspects of the spinal cord can be monitored. Inhalational anesthetics suppress the anterior horn cells, and consequently their use makes obtaining MEPs more difficult. Intravenous anesthetics (propofol and opiods) are preferred when MEP monitoring is to be used. Robust MEP responses are initially obtained from both upper (*thin arrows*) and lower (*thick arrows*) extremities in the above examples, and maintained throughout the case with similarly robust upper (*dashed arrows*) and lower (*dotted arrows*) extremity responses.

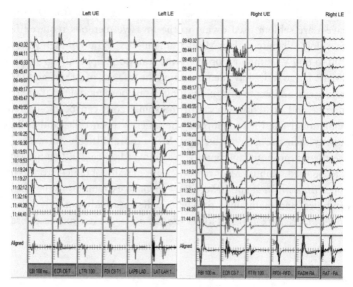

FIGURE 7.18. Intraoperative MEP monitoring showing stable responses in several upper and a single lower extremity muscle.

During surgeries in which the spinal cord is at risk, monitoring one upper and one or two lower extremity muscles is sufficient. However, in patients in whom nerve roots as well as the spinal cord is at risk (i.e., cervical stenosis/myelopathy), monitoring multiple muscles with varying root innervations may be helpful. This can allow detection of not only spinal cord injury but also injury to individual nerve roots. In the figure above, the biceps brachii (first column), extensor carpi radialis longus (*second column*), triceps (*third column*), first dorsal interosseous (*fourth column*), abductor pollicis brevis (*fifth column*), and anterior tibialis/abductor hallucis (*sixth column*) muscles are monitored in a patient undergoing multilevel cervical decompression. Robust responses are noted throughout the case, suggesting no radicular or spinal cord compromise. Notice that responses are present in alternate traces. This is because MEP stimulation can be applied selectively to one hemisphere, producing a response only on the contralateral side.

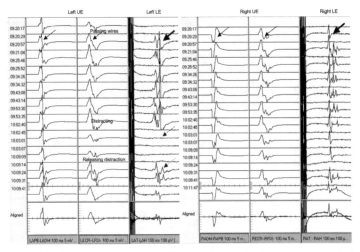

FIGURE 7.19. Intraoperative MEP monitoring during posterior spinal fusion for scoliosis showing stable responses in both upper extremities and the right lower extremity, but a transient loss of the MEP response in the left lower extremity.

Unlike BAEP and SEP, there is disagreement as to what is a significant MEP change. Some investigators suggest that a significant change occurs when the stimulus intensity has to be increased during the case to elicit the same response. Others suggest a significant change occurs only when the response is completely lost, regardless of the stimulation intensity. In the author's experience, a significant response is one in which the response disappears completely or by at least 90%. In the example above, at the start of the case MEP responses are noted in both upper (*first two columns of each graph; thin arrows*) and lower (*last column in each graph; thick arrows*) extremities. With distraction, there was loss of the left lower extremity MEP (*dashed arrow*). The surgeon was notified and the distraction was relaxed with return of the MEP (*dotted arrow*).

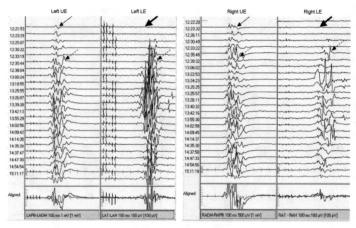

FIGURE 7.20. Intraoperative MEP monitoring in a patient undergoing spinal cord tumor biopsy showing the initial absence of the MEP responses in the lower extremities due to administration of neuromuscular blocking agents during induction and the subsequent return with drug cessation.

MEPs are very sensitive to inhalational anesthetics and neuromuscular-blocking agents. When these drugs are given in boluses (i.e., during induction), the affect on MEPs is striking. Maintaining low doses of both agents may be compatible with MEP monitoring. In the above example, initially the upper extremity MEP (*first column*) were seen (*thin arrows*), but lower extremity responses were absent (*thick arrows*) during induction with neuromuscular- blocking agents. When further boluses of neuromuscular-blocking agents were not administered, after a few minutes robust MEPs were seen for both upper and lower extremities (*dashed arrows*).

ELECTROMYOGRAPHY

When nerve roots are at risk during surgery, monitoring spontaneous and stimulated EMG provides useful information to help preserve the nerve roots. Various abnormalities can be detected with this type of NIOM and can help reduce neurologic morbidity.

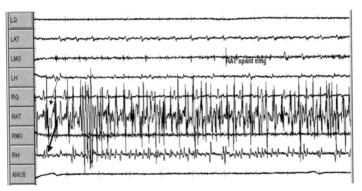

FIGURE 7.21. Intraoperative free-running EMG monitoring showing a neurotonic discharge primarily arising from the right anterior tibialis muscle (L4 to L5 root) during tethered cord release. One second is displayed.

Monitoring of the peripheral nervous system can be performed with the use of free-running EMG, stimulated EMG, or nerve action potentials. To record free-running (or stimulated) EMG, needle or wire electrodes are placed in muscles innervated by nerves that are at risk. Significant injury to nerves during dissection produces high-frequency discharges called neurotonic discharges. Short bursts of neurotonic discharges signify transient nerve injury; if persistent, the injury may be irreversible. In the figure above, the channels monitored are left vastus lateralis, left anterior tibialis, left medial gastrocnemius, left semitendinosis, right vastus lateralis, right anterior tibialis, right medial gastrocnemius, right semitendinosis, and anal sphincter muscles using needle electrodes. There is a high-frequency run of discharges consistent with a neurotonic discharge arising from the right anterior tibialis muscle (*thin arrow*) and to a lesser extent from the right hamstring muscle (*thick arrow*). Upon hearing the discharge, the surgeon stopped dissecting, irrigated the surgical field, and the neuro-tonic discharge resolved.

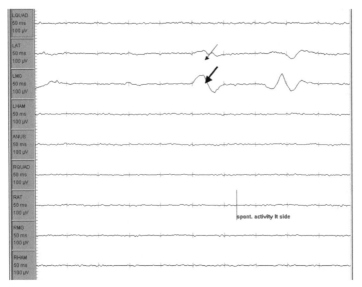

FIGURE 7.22. Intraoperative free-running EMG monitoring data showing occasional spontaneous muscle activity arising from the left anterior tibialis and medial gastrocnemius muscles. The left vastus lateralis, left anterior tibialis, left medial gastrocnemius, left semitendinosis, anal sphincter, right vastus lateralis, right anterior tibialis, right medial gastrocnemius, and right semitendinosis muscles are being monitored.

Minor irritation of a nerve often causes spontaneous firing of motor units supplied by that nerve. While monitoring free-running EMG, this is manifested as low-frequency, short discharges. These discharges are not associated with postoperative morbidity. The example above displays 50 msec of data from a patient undergoing tethered cord release surgery. During irrigation low-frequency discharges are noted in the left anterior tibialis (*thin arrow*) and medial gastrocnemius (*thick arrow*) muscles that disappeared after a few seconds.

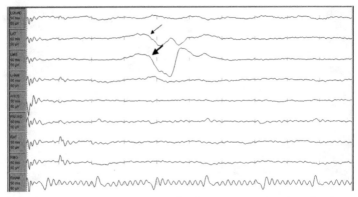

FIGURE 7.23. Intraoperative stimulated EMG monitoring data showing a response in the left anterior tibialis and medial gastrocnemius muscles. This is a 100 msec sample. The montage is left vastus lateralis, left anterior tibialis, left medial gastrocnemius, left semitendinosis, anal sphincter, right vastus lateralis, right anterior tibialis, right medial gastrocnemius, and right semitendinosis muscles.

Stimulated EMG can be used to identify neural structures during surgery. For example, if a tumor is surrounding neural tissue, focal stimulation in various areas of the tumor can be helpful in determining where neural elements are present. Alternatively, often when anatomy is not clear, structures in the surgical field can be stimulated, and according to the pattern of response seen, they can be correctly identified. In the figure above, stimulation of a nerve root produced a triggered response in the left anterior tibialis (*thin arrow*) and the medial gastrocnemius (*thick arrow*) muscles. The root stimulated is most likely the left L5 root.

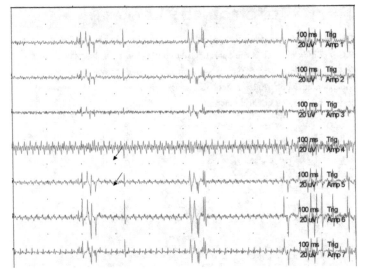

FIGURE 7.24. Intraoperative EMG monitoring data showing an artifact that resembles a neurotonic discharge. One second is displayed. The montage is left anterior tibialis, left medial gastrocnemius, left semitendinosis, anal sphincter, right anterior tibialis, right medial gastrocnemius, and right semitendinosis muscles.

As with other types of monitoring, artifacts are common in EMG monitoring as well. Differentiating artifacts from neurotonic discharges is critical to avoid unnecessary surgical intervention. In the figure above, the patient is undergoing tethered cord release surgery. Although runs of high-frequency discharges are seen, they are not neurotonic discharges. Their widespread, rhythmic, and similar morphology in all channels (*arrows*) provides proper identification as artifact.

ELECTROENCEPHALOGRAPHY

The EEG may demonstrate changes as a reflection of cerebral blood flow. Therefore, EEG is commonly used in the operating suite during surgeries that may impair blood flow to the brain. The EEG may also be useful to directly record epileptiform, nonepileptiform, or evoked potentials during surgical resections that require identification of eloquent cortical function.

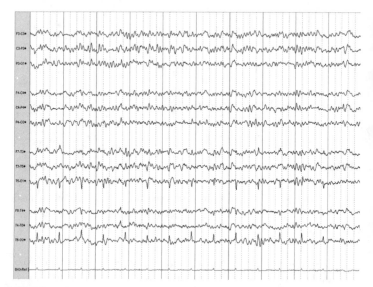

FIGURE 7.25. Intraoperative EEG during right carotid endarterectomy demonstrating bilateral symmetrical cerebral activity after clamping of the right carotid artery. The montage is a longitudinal bipolar montage (left over right; parasagital over temporal). The Fp1 and Fp2 electrodes were not applied because of anesthesia monitor placement in that location.

EEG monitoring is often used when the vascular supply to the brain may be interrupted. Carotid endarterectomy (CEA) is a common indication for such monitoring. During CEA, if slowing is noted ipsilateral to the side of clamping of the carotid artery, bypass (shunting) procedures are considered. If slowing or voltage reduction is seen over the ipsilateral hemisphere, it usually occurs within a minute after clamping. No changes in the EEG implies adequate collateral perfusion. The preceeding example (Figure 7.25) is a 10-sec sample taken several minutes after clamping the carotid artery. The EEG continued to look bilaterally symmetrical, implying adequate collateral circulation.

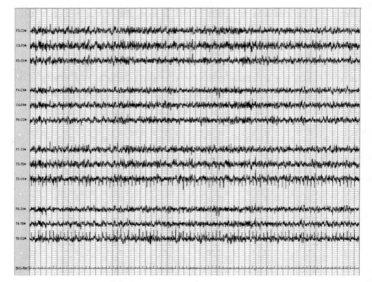

FIGURE 7.26. Intraoperative EEG taken from the same patient as in the last figure. A 60-sec page is displayed. Note the bilaterally symmetric activity.

When monitoring EEG during CEA, often a slower (60 sec) display is useful to accentuate asymmetrical slowing and/or loss of faster frequencies.

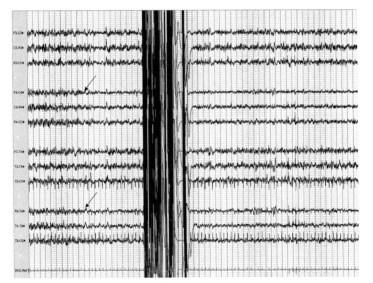

FIGURE 7.27. Intraoperative EEG showing loss of faster frequencies over the right hemisphere after clamping of the right carotid artery.

As noted previously, slower visual displays (paper speed) can be helpful in identifying slowing and loss of faster frequencies. When slowing occurs during clamping of the carotid artery, shunt placement to bypass the iatrogenicly induced ischemia is considered. The example shown above was taken from a patient that was undergoing a right CEA, and approximately 1 min after clamping the right carotid artery, there was a loss of faster frequencies in that hemisphere (*arrows*). The clamp was removed, the EEG returned to baseline, and no postoperative deficit was incurred.

ADDITIONAL RESOURCES

James ML, Husain AM. Brainstem auditory evoked potential monitoring: when is change in wave V significant? *Neurology* 2005;65(10):1551-1555.

Legatt AD. Mechanisms of intraoperative brainstem auditory evoked potential changes. *J Clin Neurophysiol* 2002;19(5):396–408.

MacDonald DB. Safety of intraoperative transcranial electrical stimulation motor evoked potential monitoring. *J Clin Neurophysiol* 2002;19(5): 416–429.

Nuwer MR, Dawson EG, Carlson LG, et al. Somatosensory evoked potential spinal cord monitoring reduces neurologic deficits after scoliosis surgery: results of a large multicenter survey. *Electroencephalogr Clin Neurophysiol* 1995;96(1):6–11.

Radtke RA, Erwin CW, Wilkins RH. Intraoperative brainstem auditory evoked potentials: significant decrease in postoperative morbidity. *Neurology* 1989;39(2 Pt 1):187–191.

Robertson SC, Traynelis VC, Yamada TT. Identification of the sensorimotor cortex with SSEP phase reversal. In: Loftus CM, and Traynelis VC, eds. *Intraoperative Monitoring Techniques in Neurosurgery.* McGraw-Hill, New York, 1994:107–111.

Seyal M, Mull B. Mechanisms of signal change during intraoperative somatosensory evoked potential monitoring of the spinal cord. *J Clin Neurophysiol* 2002;19(5):409–415.

Index